# Yoga for Arthritis

## Best Yoga Poses to Reduce Inflammation Pain, Increase Strength, Balance, and Flexibility

Noah Miller

**Copyrights**

All rights reserved © 2017 by Noah Miller. No part of this publication or the information in it may be quoted from or reproduced in any form by means such as printing, scanning, photocopying, or otherwise without prior written permission of the copyright holder.

**Disclaimer and Terms of Use**

Efforts has been made to ensure that the information in this book is accurate and complete. However, the author and the publisher do not warrant the accuracy of the information, text, and graphics contained within the book due to the rapidly changing nature of science, research, known and unknown facts, and internet. The author and the publisher do not hold any responsibility for errors, omissions, or contrary interpretation of the subject matter herein. This book is presented solely for motivational and informational purposes only

**ISBN: 978-1986511704**

**Printed in the United States**

# Contents

Introduction ........................................................................................... 1
The Benefits of Yoga ............................................................................. 3
Yoga for Arthritis .................................................................................... 7
Shoulder Pain ........................................................................................ 7
    Eagle Arms ....................................................................................... 7
    Thread the Needle ........................................................................... 9
    Low Lunge Twist Pose ................................................................... 11
    Sanskrit name: Parivrtta Sanchalasana ....................................... 11
    Cow Face Pose .............................................................................. 13
    Bharadvaja's Twist ......................................................................... 15
    Standing Forward Fold with Hand Clasp ..................................... 17
    Reverse Prayer Hands ................................................................... 19
Back Pain ............................................................................................. 21
    Supported Bridge Pose ................................................................. 21
    Supine Twisting Posture ............................................................... 23
    Cobra Pose ..................................................................................... 25
    Sphinx Pose ................................................................................... 27
    Melting Heart Posture ................................................................... 29
    Rabbit Pose .................................................................................... 31
    Half Lord of the Fishes Pose ........................................................ 33
    Tree Pose ....................................................................................... 35
Hip Relief ............................................................................................. 37
    Low Lunge ..................................................................................... 37
    High Lunge .................................................................................... 39
    Warrior I Pose ................................................................................ 41
    Goddess Pose ............................................................................... 43
    Reclining Pigeon Pose .................................................................. 45
    Restorative Child's Pose ............................................................... 47
    Happy Baby Pose .......................................................................... 49
    Fire Log Pose ................................................................................. 51
    Lizard Pose .................................................................................... 53
Knee Pain ............................................................................................. 55
    Wide Angle Seated Forward Bend ............................................... 55
    Standing Figure Four .................................................................... 57
    Warrior II Pose ............................................................................... 59
    Modified Bound Angle Pose ......................................................... 61
    Modified Garland Pose ................................................................. 63
    Extended Triangle Pose ................................................................ 65
    Modified Easy Pose ...................................................................... 67
    Half Moon Pose ............................................................................. 69
    Supported Reclining Hero Pose ................................................... 71
    Lotus Pose ..................................................................................... 73

## Releasing the Neck — 75
### Downward Facing Dog — 75
### Wide Legged Standing Forward Bend — 77
### Modified Fish Pose — 79
### Cat and Cow Poses — 81
### Rag Doll — 83
### Standing Split — 85
### Camel Pose — 87
### Dolphin Pose — 89
### Upward Plank Pose — 91

## Autoimmune Symptoms — 93
### Mountain Pose — 93
### Skull Shining Breath — 95
### Legs Up the Wall Pose — 97
### Alternate Nostril Breathing — 99
### Staff Pose — 101
### Restorative Reclining Bound Angle Pose — 103
### Corpse Pose — 105

## Parting Words and The Yoga Lifestyle — 107

# Introduction

Yoga is not just a form of exercise. When it developed in India thousands of years ago, it was intended as a path to spiritual enlightenment. In fact, the word *yoga* means "to join together." It uses poses, breathing, and meditation to unite the body and mind, and brings (among many other health benefits) a sense of peace and well-being. In yoga, mind, body, and spirit are considered three inseparable parts of the whole.

Feeling good is enough encouragement for many to participate in the practice, but if you're suffering from the chronic stiffness, pain, and discomfort of arthritis and related conditions, there is even better news: yoga can do you a world of good.

It sounds counter-intuitive. When you're in pain, you don't want to think about getting down on the floor and contorting into all those unlikely positions. But that is the *ideal* time to begin. Many poses are gentle and easy, and still deliver benefits. If you spend some time on those, soon you'll be ready for some intermediate poses. It's a process, and remember that you don't need to do any of the poses perfectly for them to help you.

Yoga is for almost everyone – just have a quick talk with your doctor if you have any concerns. After that, all you need to do is study the poses, set aside some time for yourself, and try. You will soon find your flexibility and strength increasing, and you'll start to see some of the many, many other benefits of yoga.

# The Benefits of Yoga

## Yoga for the Body

Yoga poses encourage both strength and flexibility, but because the practice honors the person as a whole, you always work at your own pace. This is what makes yoga perfect for arthritis sufferers – you perform the poses within the boundaries of your own ability and comfort. When you're starting out, you might have some muscle groups that are weak, and that's fine. Gentle effort is all that's required to begin strengthening them. You'll also have stiff places you might not even be aware of, and it's a rare treat when you find a stretch that eases them.

For arthritis sufferers, the main benefits of yoga are improved strength, flexibility, and balance. Muscle strength is important because strong muscles can help to support and take strain off the joints. Flexibility in the joints will give you a better range of motion and improve your comfort, both when you're awake and when you're trying to sleep. And balance, largely a product of the first two, means you're less likely to suffer a painful injury that will take time to heal. All of these lead to an increase in mobility, and a reduction in pain.

So yoga soothes and fortifies the body, but there are a host of other ways it helps you. The practice has been shown to improve brain function, lower blood pressure, improve circulation, and build lung capacity. Many twisting poses aid digestion, and help with bloating and discomfort caused by the continued use of painkillers.

Inflammation causes or exacerbates many health problems, including types of arthritis. While short-term or sporadic yoga practice does not help with inflammation, there is some evidence that it can help, if you're dedicated. In 2010, Janice Kiecolt-Glaser, PhD, conducted a study at Ohio State University, Columbus. She measured the levels of proteins linked with inflammation in the blood of yoga practitioners. She found that newer participants had higher levels of these proteins than those who had been doing yoga for a while; however, there were no immediate changes in these levels in the short term. She notes that the people in her study were similar in terms of age, body type, and health habits.

Whether it was the poses, the exercise, the breathing techniques, or the meditation, it's encouraging to note that the participants also reported feeling better emotionally. Yoga will sometimes relieve the pain, but even if it doesn't entirely, it does help with your frame of mind. A good outlook has been shown to decrease your *experience* of the discomfort, and give you the fortitude to withstand it better.

As we've said, yoga brings us into touch with ourselves, body, mind, and spirit. It encourages self-care, and makes us more aware of how our bodies are feeling. This awareness can lead to a change in other habits as well, such as eating healthier, or getting more sleep. These things in turn contribute to your overall health, which reduces your pain and makes you stronger in both body and mind.

## Yoga for the Mind

Yoga works on the nervous system, and it also stimulates our glands with its twisting and stretching. This is how it's able to help us feel more relaxed and at ease, reducing stress and anxiety and bringing emotional comfort as well as physical.

Part of the reason for this is that the slow, deliberate breathing techniques we use in yoga serve to distract us from the hundreds of trivial thoughts that run through our minds. When we pay closer attention to our inner self, we are able to think more clearly, and this makes us feel calmer. The more time we are able to spend in this calm state, the better able we are to detach from the external tensions affecting us.

Meditation has been shown to reduce stress, and this is especially important for people with arthritis and related conditions. Not only are you dealing with the regular problems of daily life, like bills, deadlines, appointments, and obligations, but you have an extra layer added by chronic pain. Now you're dealing with physical discomfort, loss of sleep and fatigue, physical limitations, job complications, and maybe even the loss of your independence and self-confidence.

Because of these extra physical, real-life challenges, it's especially important that people with arthritis pay particular attention to self-care, both physically and emotionally. Setting time aside for yoga will help you accomplish both.

Part of the challenge of dealing with anxiety is calming the body, because it is difficult to settle the mind when you're experiencing physical stress responses like shallow breathing, elevated heart rate, and sweating. Some people don't even realize when this is happening; they only know they feel terribly agitated. The regular practice of yoga teaches us to be self-aware and reach a state of calm more quickly and deliberately, through regulating the breath, and focusing the mind inward. Once the body begins to settle down, the mind can as well. As we have said, yoga addresses mind, body, and spirit as a whole.

## Yoga and You

As you turn through the pages of this book, you may be inspired by the poses shown, but you may feel intimidated. *Don't worry*. These pictures are intended to show what your goal might be ultimately, but in almost every pose there are modifications, helpful hints, props, and exceptions for your situation.

***Things you may want to have on hand:***
- A thick yoga mat
- Yoga blocks
- A yoga strap, or an improvised one like a scarf or belt
- A thick pillow or two
- A blanket you can fold into the desired shape

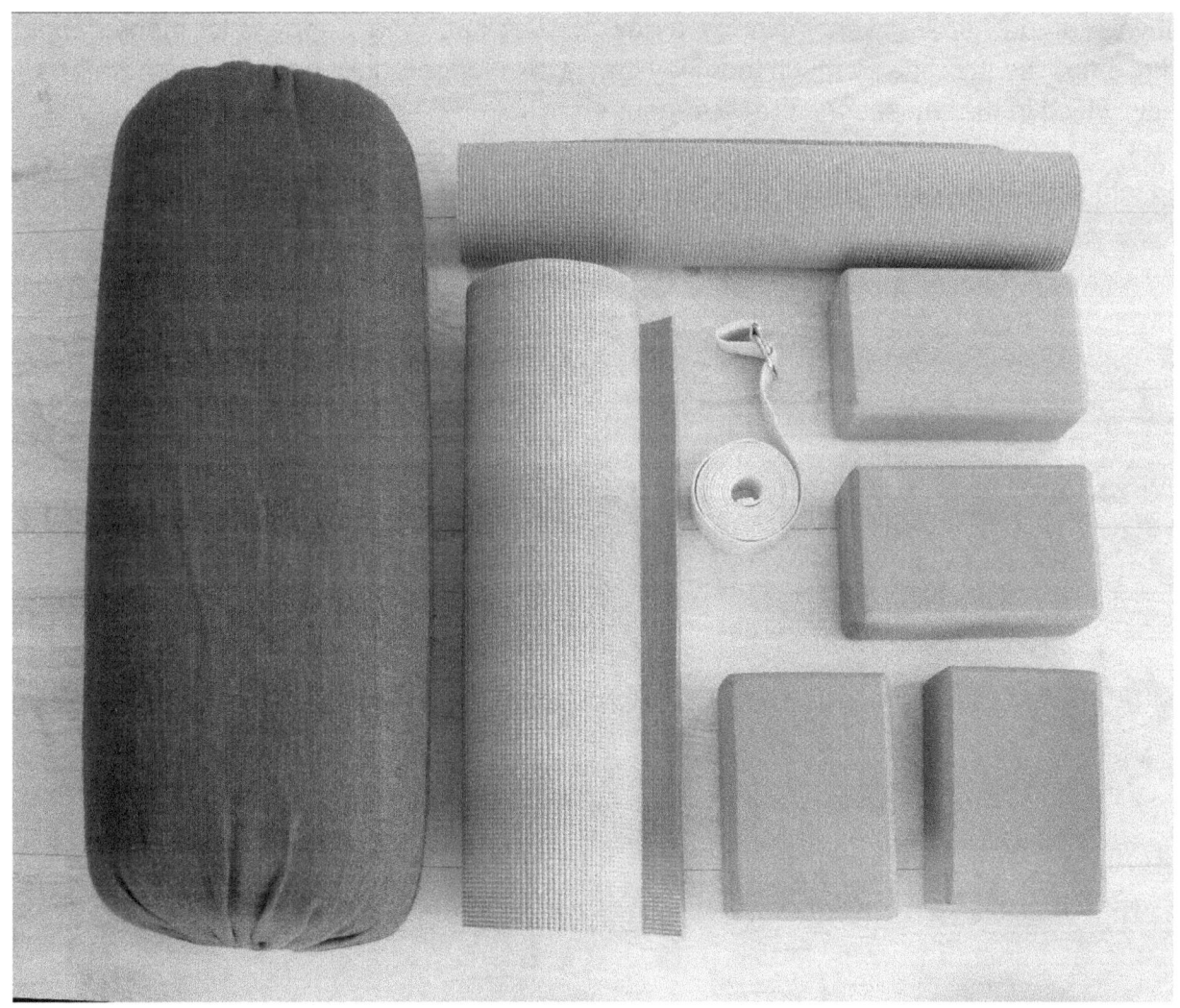

Read the instructions for the poses, and consider what your doctor or healthcare adviser has recommended. Try some of the easier poses first, always remembering to relax and breathe. The simple poses are stepping stones to the more demanding ones, and you'll be surprised how little time it takes to evolve once you've begun. You're going to feel so much better!

Some poses will feel awkward at first, and this is normal. You have not asked your body to do these things before, and even people without particular physical challenges feel strange when they begin. Do the poses the best you can, and soon you'll notice they're getting easier. Gradually, you'll build flexibility, strength, and balance.

It's natural to feel a stretch or a mild burn in your muscles, but you should never push a joint that's flaring. Any sharp pains are a signal to stop. And while you'll probably want some privacy to do your practice, keep safety in mind. Have plenty of props on hand to help you balance and do the poses. Most importantly, if your condition is severe, don't attempt difficult poses if there is nobody around to call to for help.

Are you ready to give it a try?

We can begin to form habits in as little as three weeks, and the yoga poses will start to help you even if you can only spare twenty minutes a day, starting out. What happens for many people is that they enjoy the practice so much that they stay with it longer, building more strength and flexibility, which in turn makes the practice more enjoyable.

So hop into something comfortable, take those socks off, and get started!

# Yoga for Arthritis

# Shoulder Pain

A lot of people walk around with the weight of the world on their shoulders. If you have arthritis pain in your shoulders, the tension so many people hold there might be making things even worse. One of the best tonics for shoulder tension is a massage, but many people with arthritis hesitate to get one because massages can be too painful for inflamed joints and the surrounding tissues.

Sitting behind a computer all day is especially bad for shoulder pain and arthritis because slouching over the computer creates more tension, reduces proper blood flow, and can ruin the alignment of your joints.

The poses in this section will help you to release that tension and bring a gentle stretch to sore, inflamed muscles. Building strength in the muscles of your neck and back will also help take some of the pressure off your shoulders. Regularly doing these stretches will help your joints become more flexible and give you some all-natural tools for treating and preventing pain.

## Eagle Arms

*Sanskrit name: Garudasana*

Eagle Arms is a simple pose you can add to other poses, like Chair Pose or Easy Pose, to enhance the shoulder stretch. Eagle Arms is ideal for when you've been sitting behind a desk all day because it also opens up the upper back and forces you to sit up straight, rather than slouch. Don't forget to do both sides, to keep things balanced.

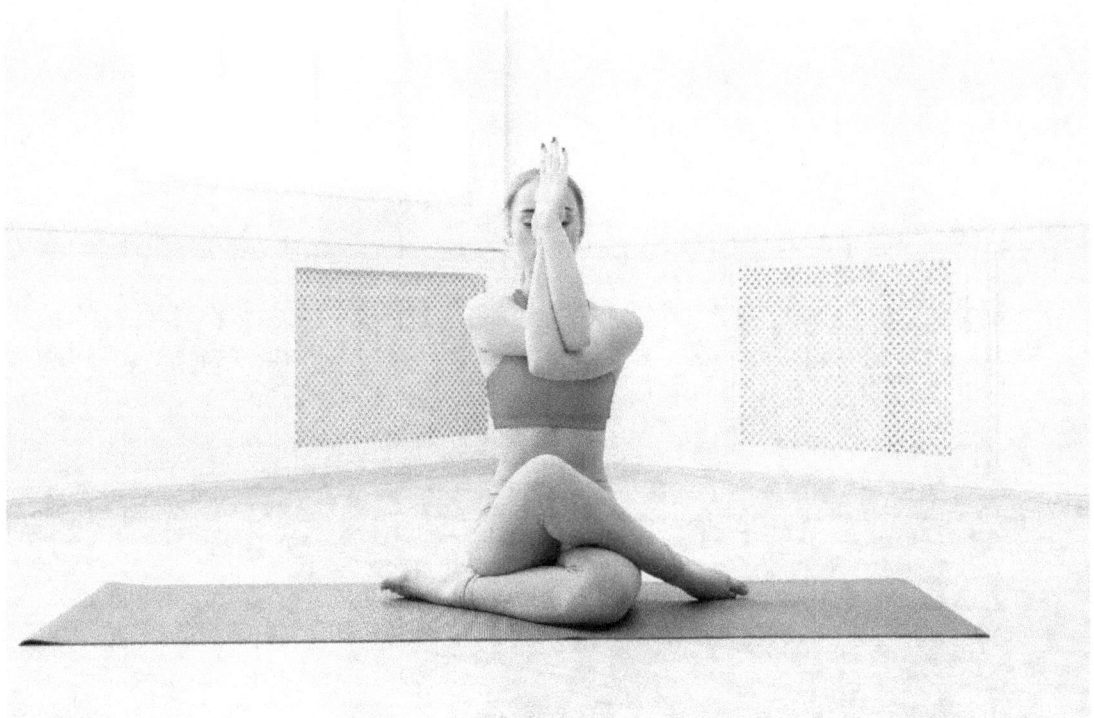

***Instructions***

1. Stretch your arms out in front of you and make sure your shoulders are relaxed. Don't allow them to creep up towards your ears.
2. Cross your left elbow over your right elbow and lift your forearms up towards your face at a 90-degree angle.
3. Turn your arms inward and try to touch your palms together.
4. Lift your arms up towards your face to the degree of your comfort. You should feel a stretch across your shoulders and upper back, but if there is any pain, stop immediately.
5. Hold the pose for 10 breaths, or as long as you can. Don't worry if your form is not perfect, as long as the stretching sensation is comfortable.
6. Repeat on the other side, crossing your right arm over the left this time.

# Thread the Needle

*Sanskrit name: Sucirandhrasana*

Thread the Needle Pose is a powerful shoulder stretch. It also opens up the chest, which corrects the harmful effects of poor posture on your neck, upper back, and shoulders.

Thread the Needle is not just a great stretch for the shoulders, back, and chest, it's also deeply calming for the central nervous system, which helps to reduce stress and manage pain. Thread the Needle is ideal any time you need a five-minute break, or when arthritis pain and stress are keeping you up at night. If you're finding your arthritis pain hard to manage, a few deep breaths in this pose can have a calming effect, while taking your mind off of the pain.

As well as stretching and aligning your upper body, Thread the Needle is also a twist posture. Twists are said to literally wring out your organs, releasing toxins and stimulating your digestive system. Many people with rheumatoid arthritis end up having to take heavy duty painkillers. This pose could be a great addition to your day to help deal with the digestive side effects of painkiller use.

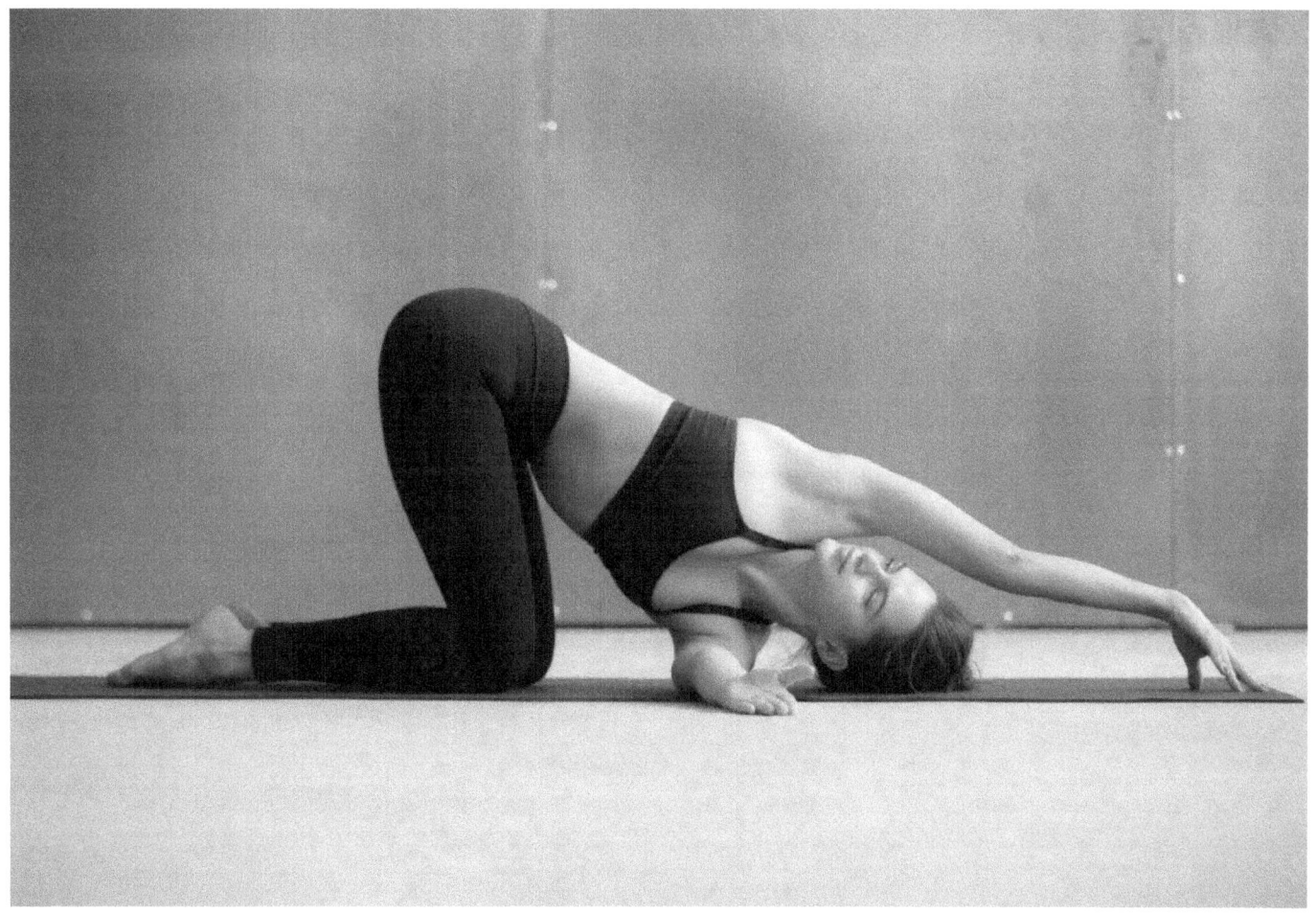

*Instructions*
1. Assume tabletop position, on your hands and knees.
2. Reach your right arm upwards towards the sky, opening your entire side body. Make sure your shoulders are stacked on top of each other, as if you were in side plank, and reach high to open up your chest.
3. Turn and thread your right arm under your left shoulder and inch it forward under your body until your right cheek and right shoulder are resting on the earth.
4. Scan your body to ensure you are holding no tension in your lower back, buttocks, or neck.
5. Take 10 deep breaths, or as many are needed to feel relief coming to your shoulders.
6. Repeat on the other side.

*Props*
1. Tabletop position requires you to rest on your knees. If you have sensitive knees, try putting a towel under them to take some of the pressure off. It's also recommended that you use a thicker mat if you have knee pain.

*Modifications*
1. If you are pregnant or have severe arthritic knee or wrist pain, you can practice this pose standing up against the wall instead.

# Low Lunge Twist Pose

*Sanskrit name: Parivrtta Sanchalasana*

Low Lunge Twist will help you to open the shoulders, chest, and hips. It will also help to develop strength and flexibility in your shoulders. However, this pose is slightly more advanced and should not be the first pose you do during your practice if you are dealing with shoulder pain. Work your way up to this pose instead, and don't continue if you feel any shooting pains.

Like Thread the Needle, Low Lunge Twist also offers the gentle twisting element that provides the detoxification and relaxation that is so calming for the digestive system, great for those on heavy medications and painkillers.

Interested in the spiritual side of yoga? This pose is said to stimulate energy and open up the heart chakra.

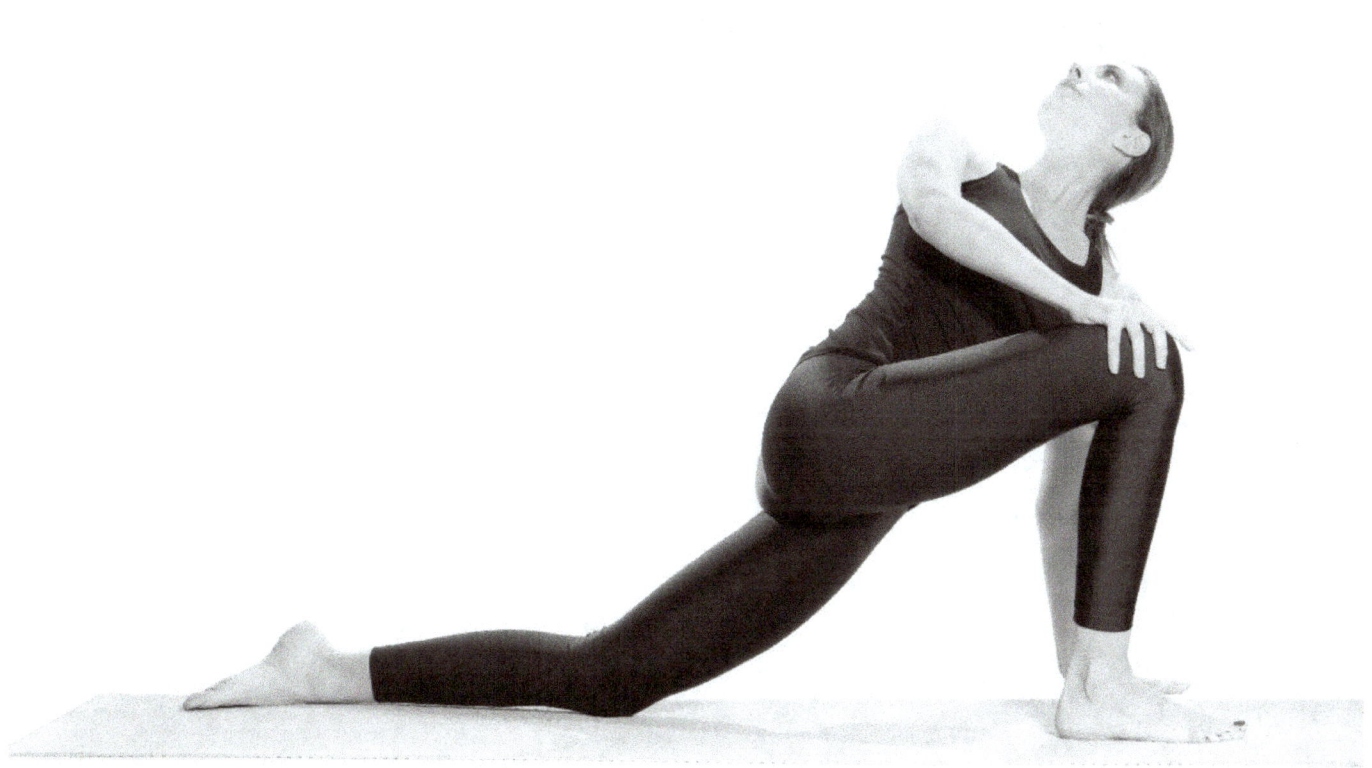

*Instructions*
1. Begin in lunge pose with your right leg forward and bent at a 90-degree angle.
2. Lower your left knee to the ground.
3. Slowly twist your entire upper body to the right.
4. From here, you can put your left hand down on the ground and rest your right hand on your knee or lift your right arm skywards.
5. Take at least five breaths, or rest here as long as needed.
6. Switch sides and repeat. You can transition through Downward Dog if desired.

*Props*
1. This pose calls for you to rest on your knees, so you might want a towel or thicker mat to prevent putting too much pressure on your knees. You can also purchase non-slip gel knee pads made specifically for yoga for around $15.00.
2. If your shoulders are too tight for your hand to reach the ground, try putting a yoga block beneath your hand.

*Modifications*
1. If you are not comfortable putting pressure on your shoulders in this pose, you may add a balancing element, which will make the pose slightly more difficult but will protect your shoulders. Instead of resting on your hand, bring your hands together in prayer pose and rest the back of your left arm on the outside of your right leg.

# Cow Face Pose

*Sanskrit name: Gomukhasana*

Cow Face Pose brings flexibility and strength to the back and shoulders, helping to reduce soreness. It also stretches out your hips. Cow Face Pose can be pretty intense on your shoulders and hips, but if you find it's too much, don't worry. Props can be used to make it much easier. Remember, strength and flexibility come with repetition, so perform the pose only to the degree that it is comfortable.

From a spiritual perspective, this pose opens the heart and sacral chakra.

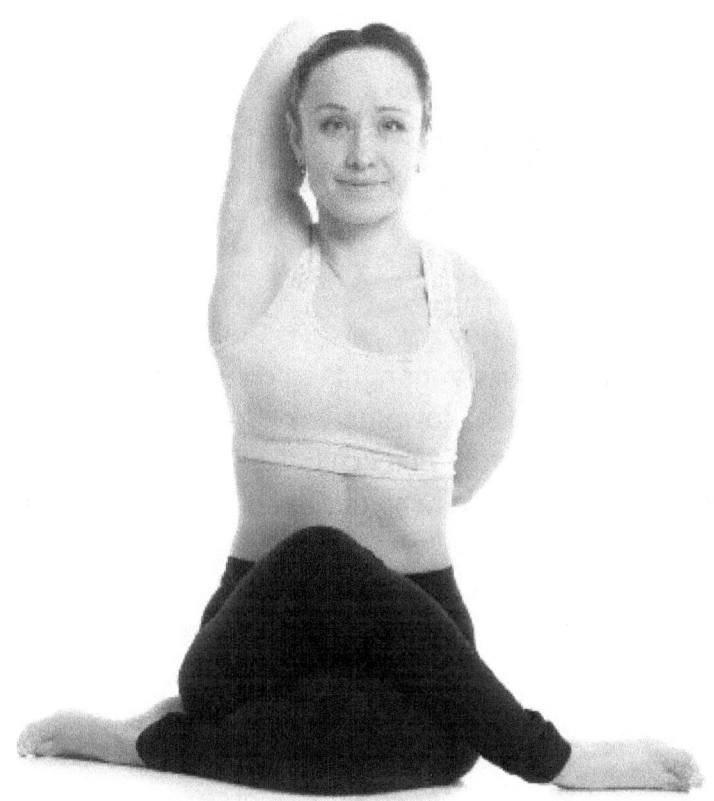

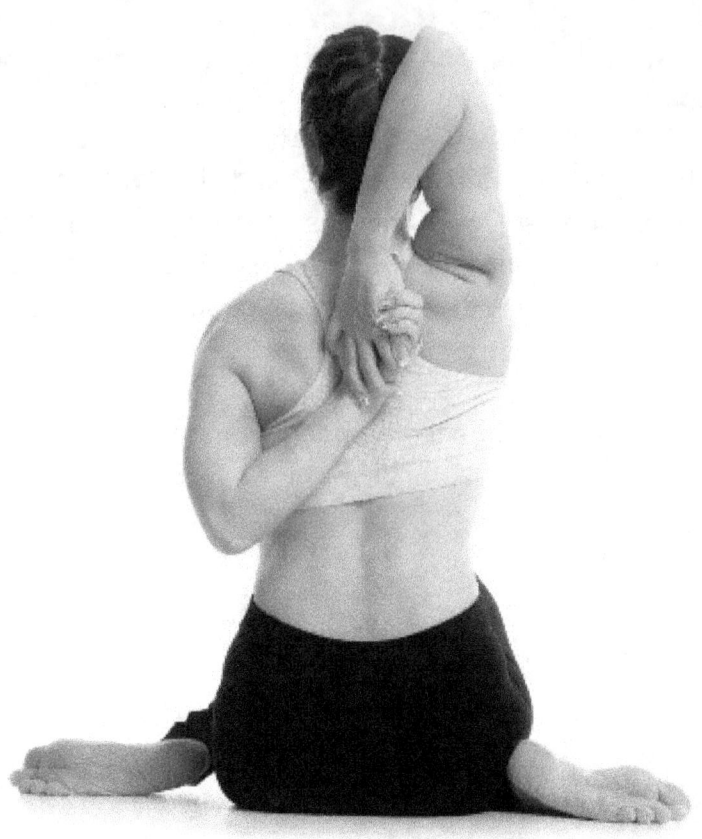

## Instructions
1. Begin seated on the ground. Cross your right leg over your left with your right knee on top of your left knee. Bend your lower legs towards your body so they cross at the knee, and the opposite foot is on either side of your body with the sole facing towards you.
2. Bend your right arm behind you and inch your hand up the center of your back.
3. Bend your left arm over your left shoulder and inch your left hand down the center of your back.
4. Try to touch your hands together, or better yet, grasp each other.
5. Breathe in this pose for about a minute, then switch sides.

## Props
1. If you are not able to touch your hands together, loop a yoga strap or hand towel between your hands, and grasp that instead.

## Modifications
1. The hip stretch this pose delivers is intense, which is a good thing, but might be too much if you're dealing with a hip injury or arthritis pain. Instead, you can skip the leg posture and focus on the shoulder stretch. Perform the arm posture while sitting erect in a chair, or on a meditation cushion.

# Bharadvaja's Twist

*Sanskrit name: Bharadvajasana*

This pose is named for Bharadvaja, a legendary seer in Hindu tradition. This pose is just as powerful as the seer!

Bharadvaja's Twist brings all the benefits of a twist while broadening your chest and opening your shoulders. It also forces you to sit up straight and brings some much-needed tension relief to your spine. This deeply grounding and relaxing pose is perfect to do before bed.

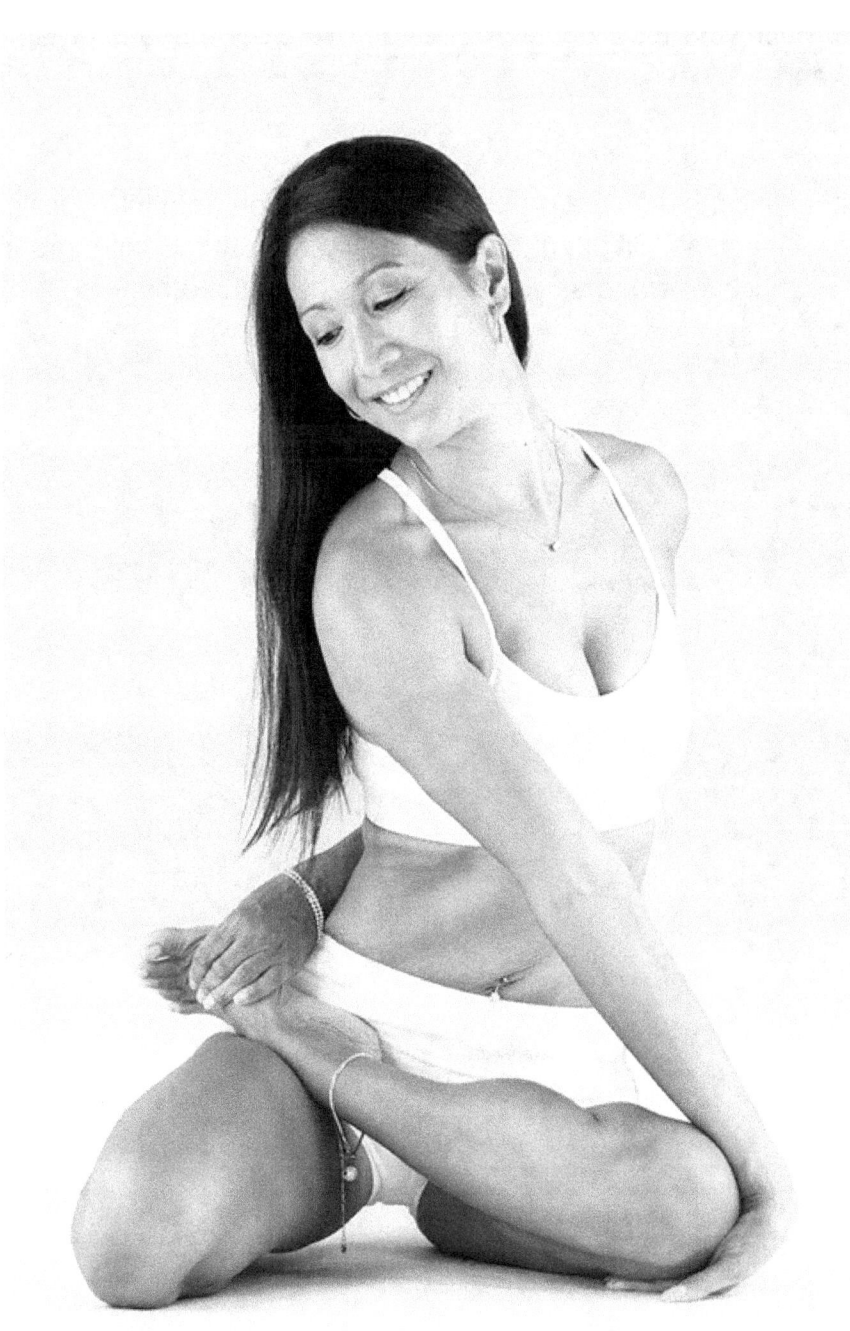

## Instructions
1. Begin seated upright on the floor with your legs out in front of you.
2. Swing your legs to the right so that both feet are sitting on the outside of your right hip. Then lift your left foot up and move it into the crease of your right hip.
3. Twist your entire upper body to the left, moving your left hand around your back to grasp your left foot.
4. Use your right arm to encourage the twist by pressing against your left leg.
5. Inhale deeply to feel the chest and shoulders opening. Breathe in this pose for 30 seconds to one minute.
6. Slowly unwind from the pose and repeat on the other side.

## Props
1. If you cannot reach your foot, loop a yoga strap over your foot and grasp it with the appropriate hand.

## Modifications
1. Instead of doing this pose on the ground and moving your foot into your hip arch, you can drop this part of the pose. Sit upright in a chair and twist to the right, grasping the back of the chair for as much leverage as you need. Repeat on the other side.

# Standing Forward Fold with Hand Clasp

*Sanskrit name: Uttānāsana*

Forward folds are soothing poses that help to release stress from the neck and shoulders. If you're holding tension in this area, it's probably making your arthritis pain even worse. This particular fold adds in the hand clasp modification to create even more of a stretch for your shoulders. Standing Forward Fold is also great for insomnia, sore hamstrings, and calming the central nervous system.

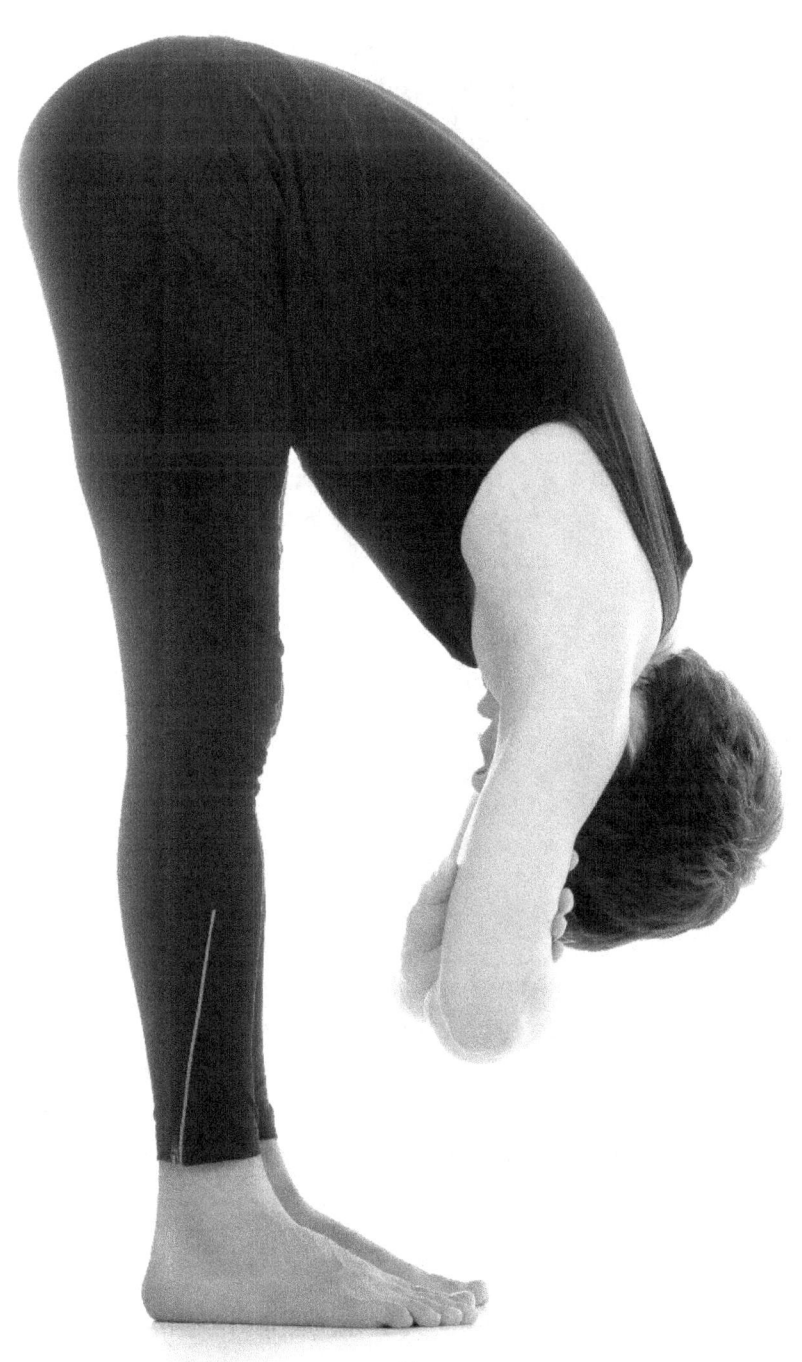

*Instructions*
1. Begin standing upright in Mountain Pose.
2. Exhale as you bend at the hips and allow your head and arms to dangle towards the ground, relaxing your neck. If you like, you can grasp your elbows with your hands to help open the shoulders.
3. Breath in this pose for as long as you need to relax and feel your shoulders and neck release tension.

## Variation for a more challenging pose

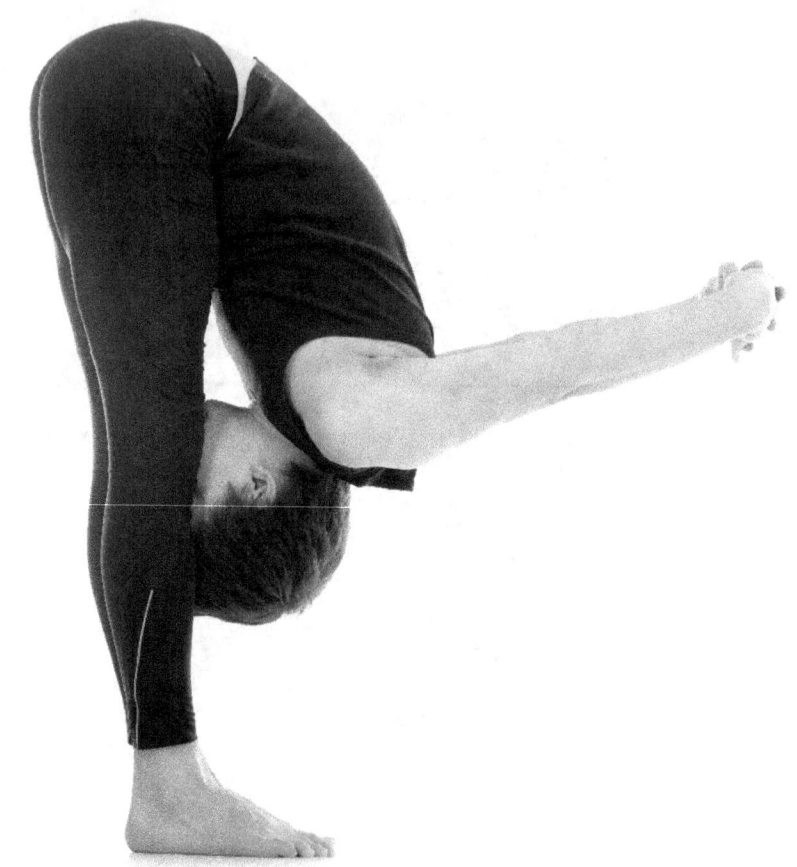

*Instructions*
1. Begin standing upright in Mountain Pose. Clasp your hands behind your back and pull them downwards, forcing your back to arch and your chest to open. Inhale deeply.
2. Exhale as you bend at the hips and allow your head to dangle towards the ground, relaxing your neck. Lift your clasped hands over your head to feel the shoulder stretch.
3. Breath in this pose for as long as you need to relax and feel your shoulders and neck release tension.

*Modifications*
1. If you have knee pain or tight hamstrings, bend your knees until your chest is resting against your thighs. This will create a more relaxing posture.

# Reverse Prayer Hands

*Sanskrit name: Pashchima Namaskarasana*

Reverse Prayer Hands delivers an intense stretch that isn't accessible for many people, even those you don't have arthritis. However, it is a powerful pose to have in your arthritis tool box if you're capable of working your way up to it.

This may be an intermediate pose, but there's lots of good news too! Reverse Prayer Hands brings tons of relief to sore wrists and fingers, spots often hit hard by arthritis that few exercises other than yoga can help. Not only does it open the chest and upper back, it also opens the heart chakra while correcting your posture.

Once you master this pose, you can add it into virtually any other posture. Add Reverse Prayer Hands to lunges, Warrior II, Easy Pose, forward folds, and more!

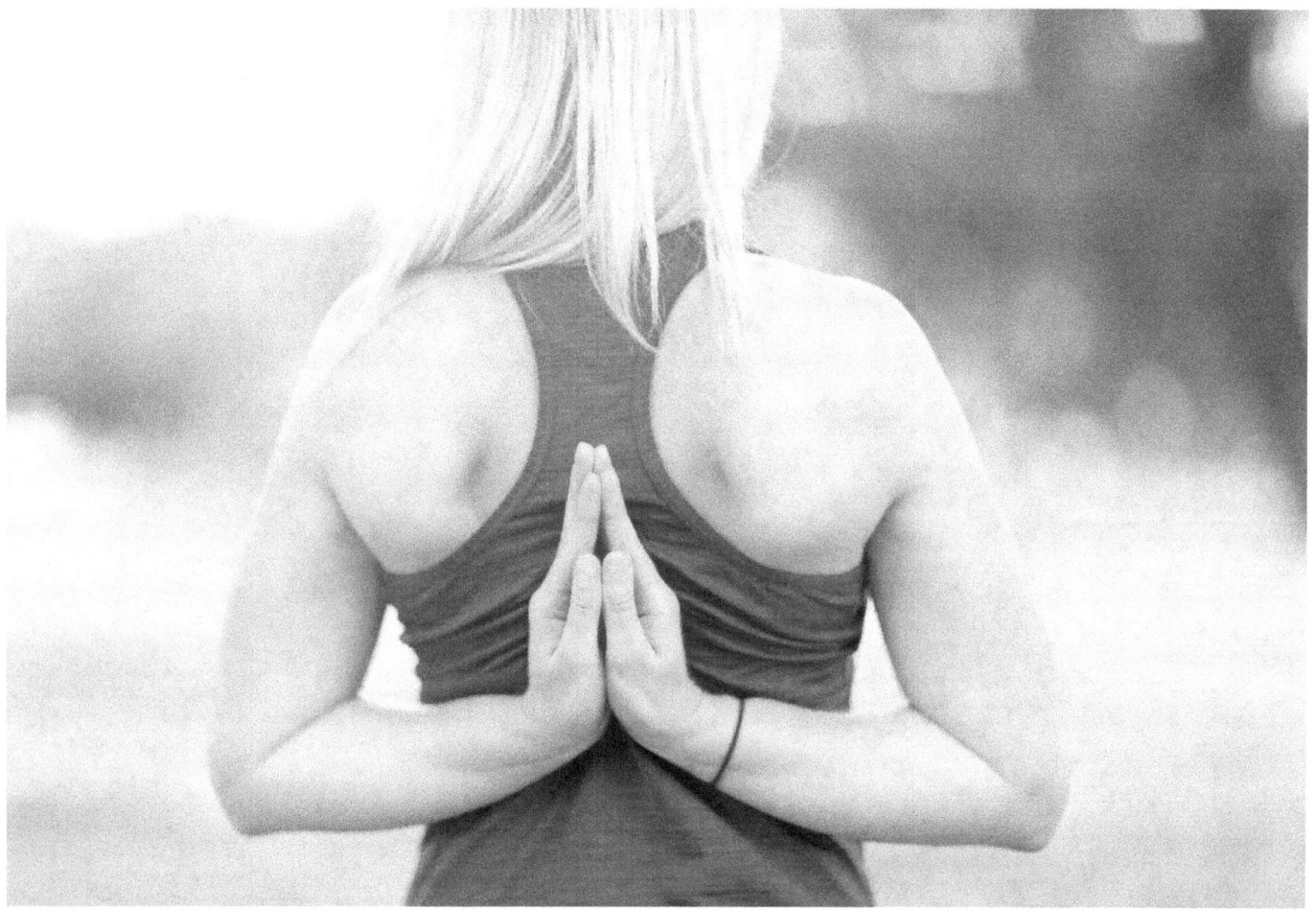

### Instructions
1. Stand upright in Mountain Pose.
2. Stretch your arms behind you and arch your back.
3. Point your fingertips upwards and bring your hands together against your back.
4. The goal is to bring your palms together as if you were praying and to move your hands up to the center of your back, ideally between the shoulder blades.
5. Breathe and hold the posture as long as needed.

### Modifications
1. Getting your palms to touch and move up to your shoulder blades just isn't going to be possible right away. Instead, start with your hands lower down on your back and focus on getting your fingertips to touch first.
2. If even that is too intense, lay one hand on your lower back and the other on top. Inhale to open your chest.

# Back Pain

Our modern, sedentary lifestyle has made back pain a fact of life. Slouching and sitting behind a desk all day make back pain so much worse. For those suffering from arthritis and osteoporosis, which often go hand in hand, treating back pain is absolutely necessary to living a quality, pain-free life.

The exercises in this section will help you reduce stress and tension that put even further strain on your back. They will also help you increase flexibility and build muscles that will protect and support your spine, and help prevent back pain in the future.

For those days when the pain is just too much to handle, this chapter also includes relaxing poses that will help you breathe through the pain.

## Supported Bridge Pose

*Sanskrit name: Setu Bandha Sarvangasana*

Supported Bridge is one of the most calming poses in the yoga canon. It's a modification of traditional Bridge Pose, and a prep for Wheel Pose. Supported Bridge is the perfect pose for opening up the hips and back, which have taken a beating from hunching over a computer or desk all day. Adding a block or cushion allows your front hips and lower back to open in a way that's just too delicious. Add this into your routine at the end of the day to help you fall asleep or unwind after work.

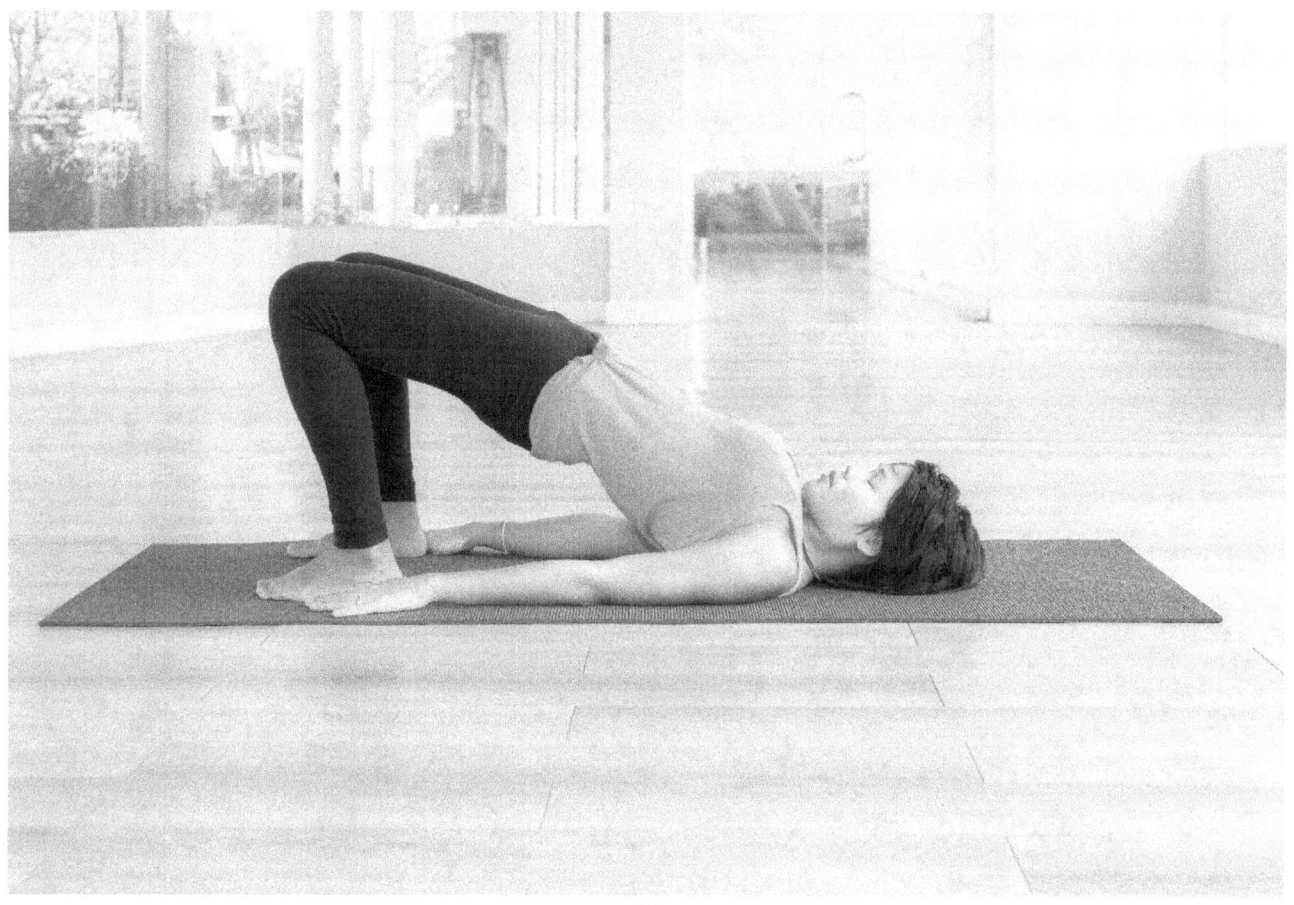

## Instructions
1. Begin by reclining on your yoga mat.
2. Bring your feet flat on the ground and move them closer to your body, creating a bend in the knees.
3. Use your leg strength to lift your buttocks a few inches off of the ground. If needed, insert the block or rolled towel beneath your sacrum (lower back) and adjust until it is comfortable.
4. Breathe, and allow gravity to stretch your hips and lower back.

## Props
1. This pose calls for a yoga block, rolled towel, or cushion. You can also use a towel or blanket under your head if your head hurts on the ground, but do not elevate your head enough to cause any strain in the neck.
2. Another option is to balance on a yoga bolster. Place the bolster vertically down your spine and relax.

# Supine Twisting Posture

*Sanskrit name: Jathara Parivartanasana*

Supine Twist is a gentle pose that's perfect for beginners. It's also one of the poses that is deeply calming for the central nervous system, making it a great way to wind down at the end of the day.

This pose is very grounding because your entire body is touching the earth, so if you're feeling jittery or flighty, add this pose into your routine. Plus, it's a twist, which means it's detoxifying and can help with any digestive symptoms you may be suffering from thanks to autoimmune disease or painkillers.

When it comes to arthritis, you might hear some glorious back cracking when you enter this posture. This pose will create space in your back where before there was just tension. Basically, all parts of your body are connected to your spine – that's why back pain is so brutal. Aligning your spine and reducing tension in your lower back can go a long way to reducing chronic pain all over your body. As an added bonus, this pose will also bring a stretch and release to your shoulders, another body part often hit hard by arthritis.

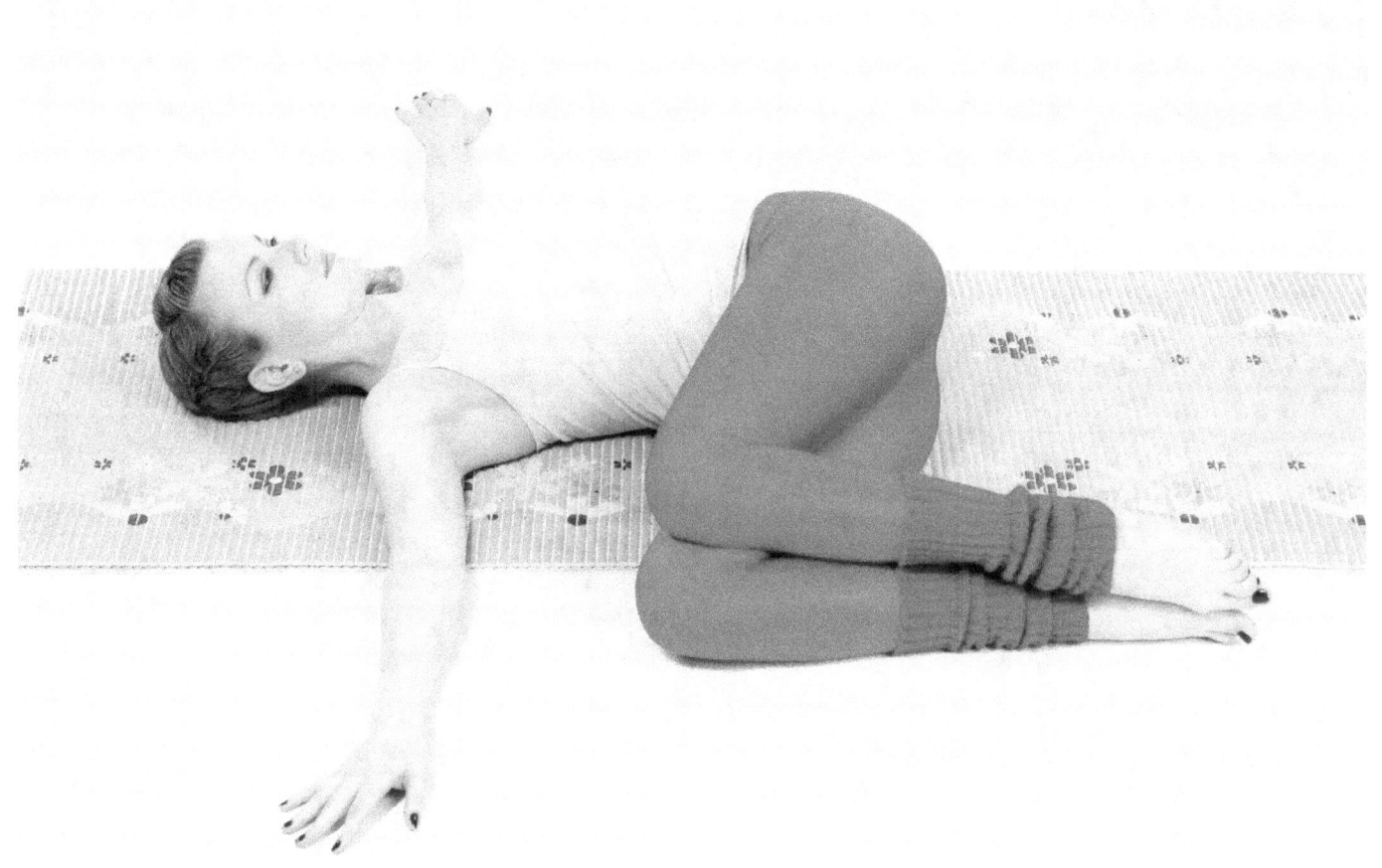

## Instructions
1. Recline on your back on your yoga mat.
2. Bring your arms out wide into a T position.
3. Bring your knees to your face, and drape them over to the right side of your body. Turn your neck to look in the opposite direction and allow gravity to work on bringing your knees to the ground.
4. To maintain the stretch to your shoulders, make sure your shoulders remain flat on the ground.
5. Breathe, and remain in this posture as long as it is comfortable.

## Props
1. This pose is simple and gentle, so it doesn't need many props. However, if your knees are sensitive, you can put a blanket beneath them.
2. If your hips are too tight for your knees to reach the floor, try placing a block beneath your knees.

## Modifications
1. If you'd like to encourage more of a stretch, place your hand on the knee to gently push it downwards towards the floor.

# Cobra Pose

*Sanskrit name: Bhujangasana*

Cobra Pose is a great transition pose during vinyasa. It serves to opens up the chest, shoulders, and back of the legs. Most importantly, it brings a stretch to your entire back, helping to reduce pain all over your body.

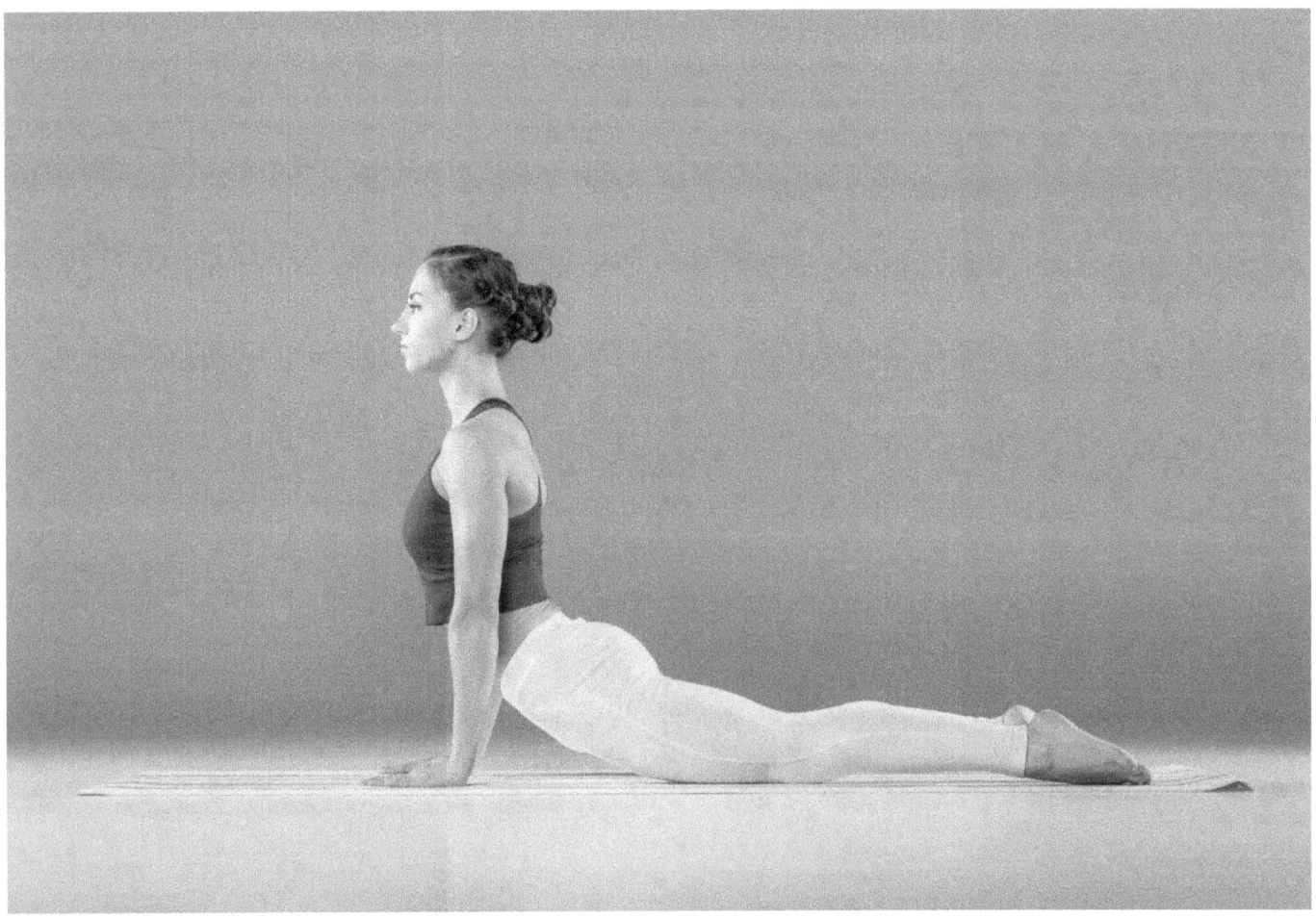

### Instructions
1. Begin by lying face down on the floor on your mat. Place your hands palms down near your shoulders.
2. Use your arm strength to lift up your chest up, while flexing your legs.
3. Inhale to open your chest. Make sure your shoulders are moving down your back, not inching their way up to your ears.
4. Take about three breaths, then release the posture.
5. Add this posture into your vinyasa or do it three times in a row for an excellent stretch to your back.

### Modifications
1. If you are too stiff and sore to lie face down on the ground, or if you are pregnant, you can do this posture standing up. Grasp the edge of a counter or a railing, and recreate the arch in your back.

# Sphinx Pose

***Sanskrit name: Salamba Bhujangasana***

If you found that Cobra Pose was too intense for you, Sphinx Pose may be what you need instead. Sphinx pose is essentially a much less intense version of Cobra Pose, making it ideal for beginners or those struggling a lot with lower back pain.

This pose stretches out your back, stomach, chest, and shoulders. Since Sphinx Pose creates a stretch across the stomach, it can also be used to treat digestive discomforts from autoimmune disorders, overeating, bloating, or painkillers.

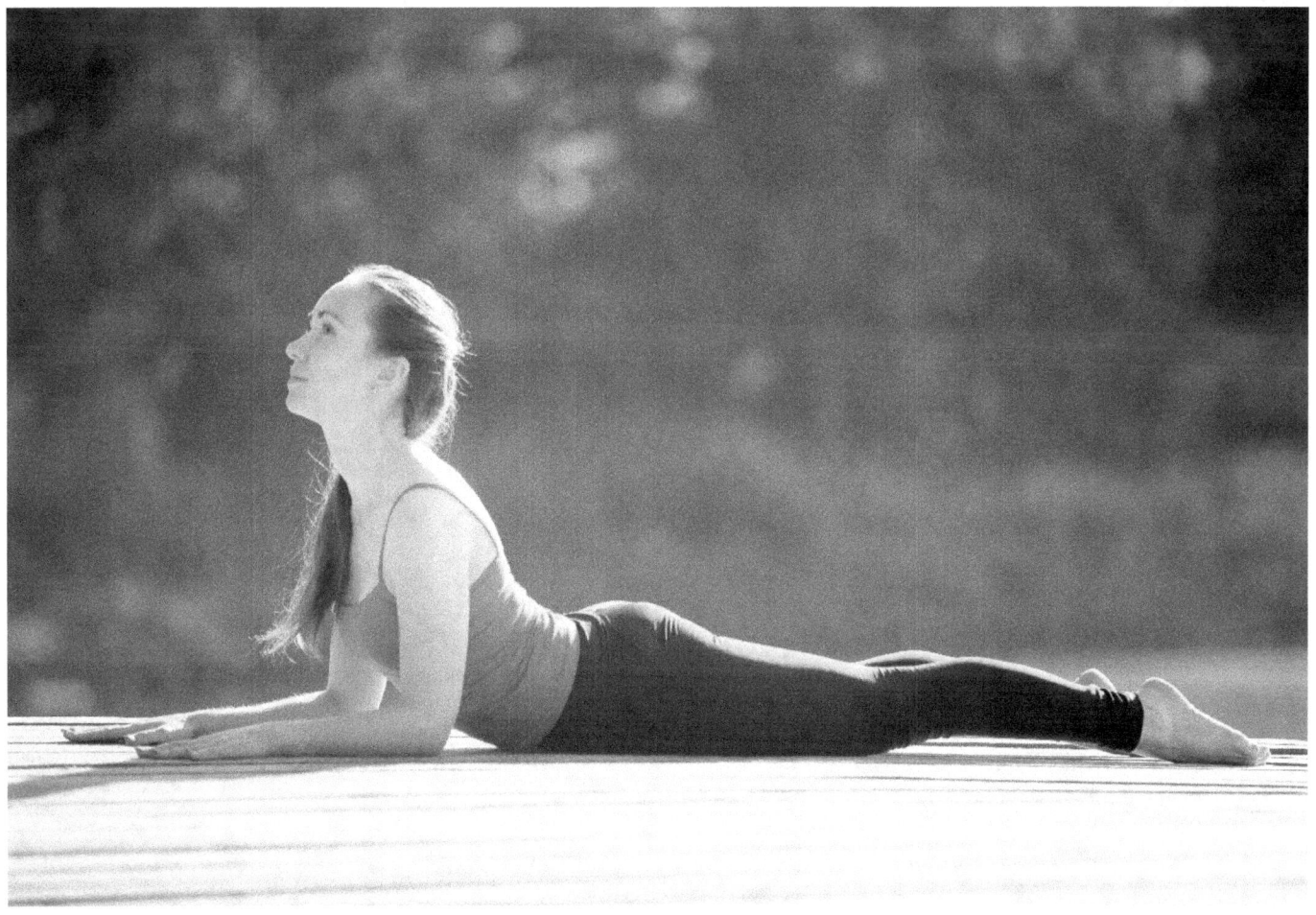

## *Instructions*
1. Begin face down on your stomach on your mat. Place your hands flat on the ground beneath each shoulder, with your forearms resting in the ground.
2. Press the tops of your feet into the ground and lift up your chest, resting on your forearms.
3. Lower your shoulders down your back, rather than allowing them to move up towards your ears.
4. Breathe deep to open the chest and remain breathing in this pose for as long as needed.

***Modifications***
1. Avoid this pose if you are pregnant or recovering from abdominal or back surgery.
2. You can also perform this pose standing up straight behind a sturdy chair or railing. Grasp the back of the chair, arch your back, and move your chest forward in the same way you would if performing this pose on the floor.

# Melting Heart Posture

*Sanskrit name: Anahatasana*

A lot of attention is paid to the lower back, and for good reason, because we tend to store tension and pain there. But since most of us sit behind a computer or the wheel of a car much more than we should, our upper and middle backs fall out of alignment and create pain for us. Melting Heart Posture, or Puppy Dog Pose, might just be the ultimate tonic for pain caused by a sedentary lifestyle.

Bad posture and a sedentary lifestyle make arthritis pain much worse, and that's why so many doctors recommend yoga. This pose will bring flexibility to a stiff back while also opening the shoulders.

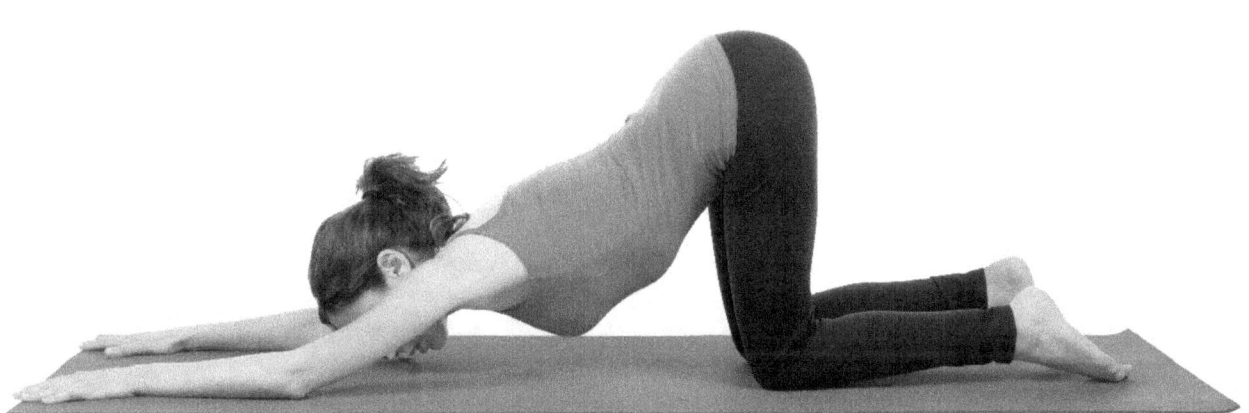

*Instructions*
1. Begin in tabletop pose, then walk your hands forward enough that your hips are still elevated while your chest is stretched towards the ground and your arms are forward.
2. While settling into the pose, feel free to move or sway the shoulders, upper body, and hips a little from side to side, for a bit of extra stretching and to find comfort and settle in.
3. Breathe while you hold this pose for up to six minutes.

## Props
1. If this pose causes too much strain or hurts your neck, place a bolster under your chest so you can rest the body.
2. This pose may not best the best choice if you have arthritis in your knees. If this is the case, use a blanket or yoga gel pads under the knees to take the pressure off.

## Modifications
1. If your shoulders are too tight, move your hands further apart.
2. For those with neck pain, this pose might put strain on the neck. If you want to relax your neck, put a bolster under your head or upper body. You can also fold one arm and rest your head on your forearm. If you choose this modification, just be sure to switch sides before ending the pose.

# Rabbit Pose

*Sanskrit name: Sasangasana*

Rabbit Pose is another brilliant way to counteract the effects of sitting behind a desk all day. This calming posture creates a stretch from your lower back through your shoulders and neck, while dissipating tension and creating space in your intervertebral discs. However, if you are dealing with a lot of neck pain or have recently had surgery, you might want to skip this posture.

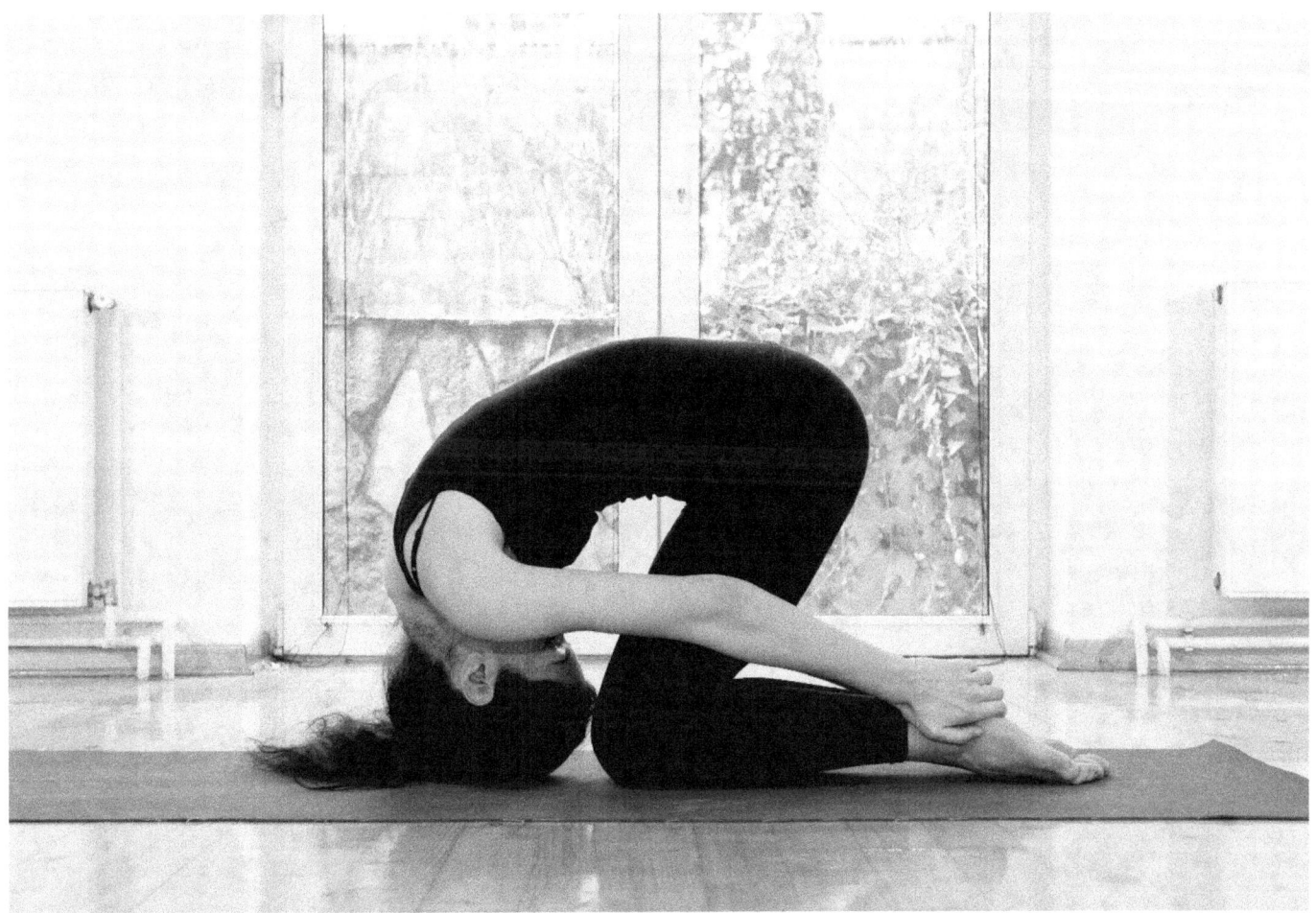

### Instructions
1. Begin by sitting on your heels. Grab your feet with your fingertips pointing inwards and your thumbs on the outside of your feet.
2. While still grasping your feet, begin to roll forward until your hips are high, your back is rounded, and the crown of your head is touching the floor. You should still be holding on to your feet.
3. Make sure your shoulders are not inching up towards your ears, and breathe for as long as needed.
4. To exit the pose, slowly shift your weight back onto your feet, and bring your back up again, one vertebrae at a time. Do not move your neck until you are sitting completely erect.

## Props
1. If you cannot reach your feet, loop a strap or a towel around your heels and hold on to that instead.
2. Since you will be resting on your knees, feel free to put a towel or a blanket under your knees.

## Modifications
1. If you'd like to intensify the shoulder stretch, add a hand clasp behind your back. This modification will, however, put greater stress on the neck.
2. Holding lower on your feet can help relieve some of the pressure on your head.

# Half Lord of the Fishes Pose

*Sanskrit name: Ardha Matsyendrasana*

Half Lord of the Fishes Pose is a gentle twist that brings relief to your lower back. It's similar to Bharadvaja's Twist, but much less intense, so if you found that twist to be too much, this pose can be a good alternative to, or even a preparation for, Bharadvaja's Twist.

This pose delivers all of the digestive benefits of a twist. It also wrings the tension out of the spine while stretching the neck, shoulders, and hips. For those who have severe back pain or have recently had back surgery, it might be best to skip this pose.

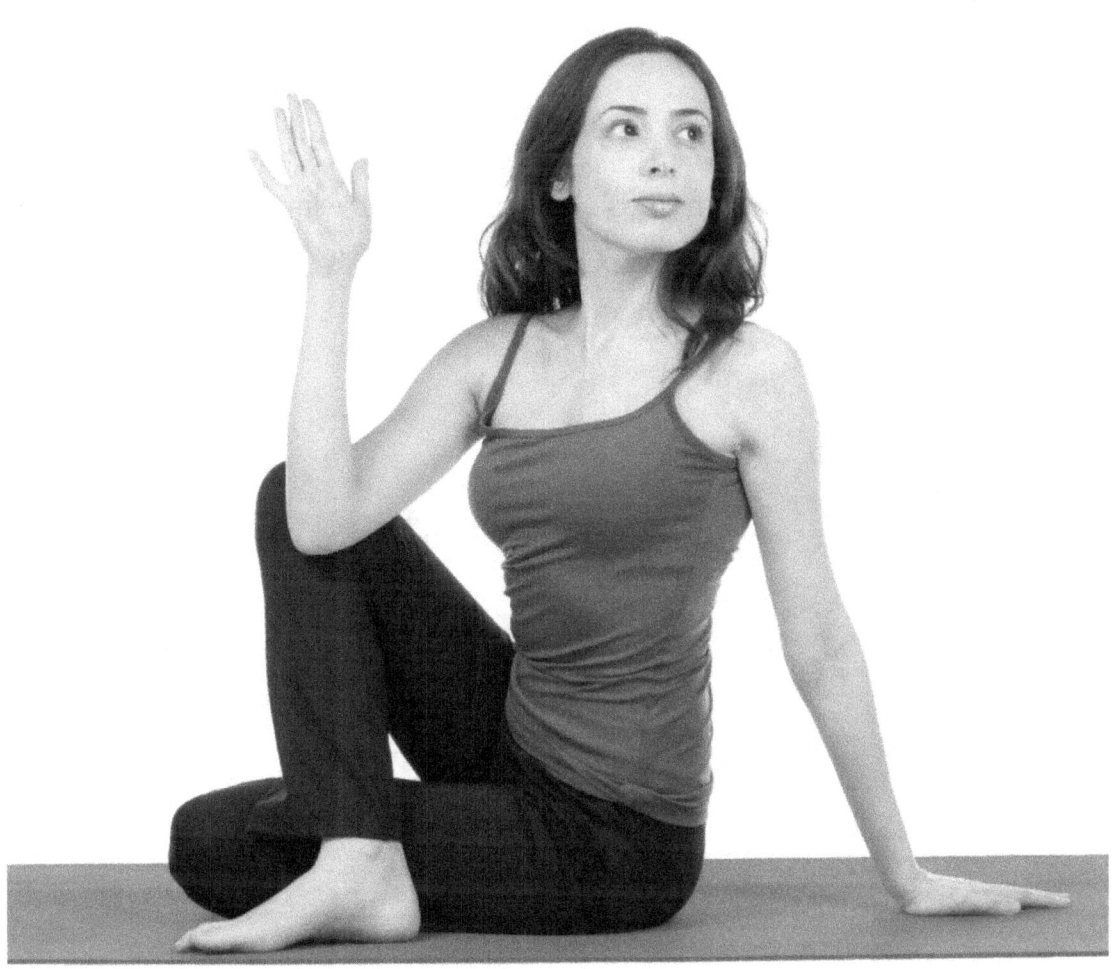

*Instructions*
1. Sit on your mat with your legs out straight in front of you, then bend your knees so your feet are flat on the ground, knees up.
2. Collapse your left leg onto the ground so your knee is still bent and your thigh is flush with the floor. Move your left foot close to your right buttock.
3. Place your right foot on the outside of your left leg, moving your left leg in closer to the body if needed.
4. Press your right arm behind your body, straight against your side, forcing you to sit upright.
5. Twist your entire upper body to the right, keeping your right arm straight. Look over your right shoulder.
6. Place your left elbow on the outside of your right leg. Your palm should be open and your hand facing upwards.
7. Breathe deeply to stretch your chest. Make sure your shoulders are moving down your back not creeping up your neck.

*Props*
1. You can also try this pose seated in a chair if your hips are tight. Grasp the back of the chair with your right hand and twist to the right. Repeat on the other side. Breathe deeply, allowing the breath to move in and out naturally with the twist.

*Modifications*
1. If you're dealing with a sore or weak back, practice this pose against the wall.
2. If your shoulders are very tight, this pose can be practiced with just the twist, leaving out the arm posture.

# Tree Pose

*Sanskrit name: Vrksasana*

One of the most important things for preventing back pain is developing strong lower back and abdominal muscles. If your arthritis is severe or you're a beginner to yoga, you might not be ready for an intense ab workout.

Balancing poses are a great alternative because they help to gently strengthen your core. Tree Pose in particular is especially helpful for those suffering from arthritis because it also opens the chest and the hips.

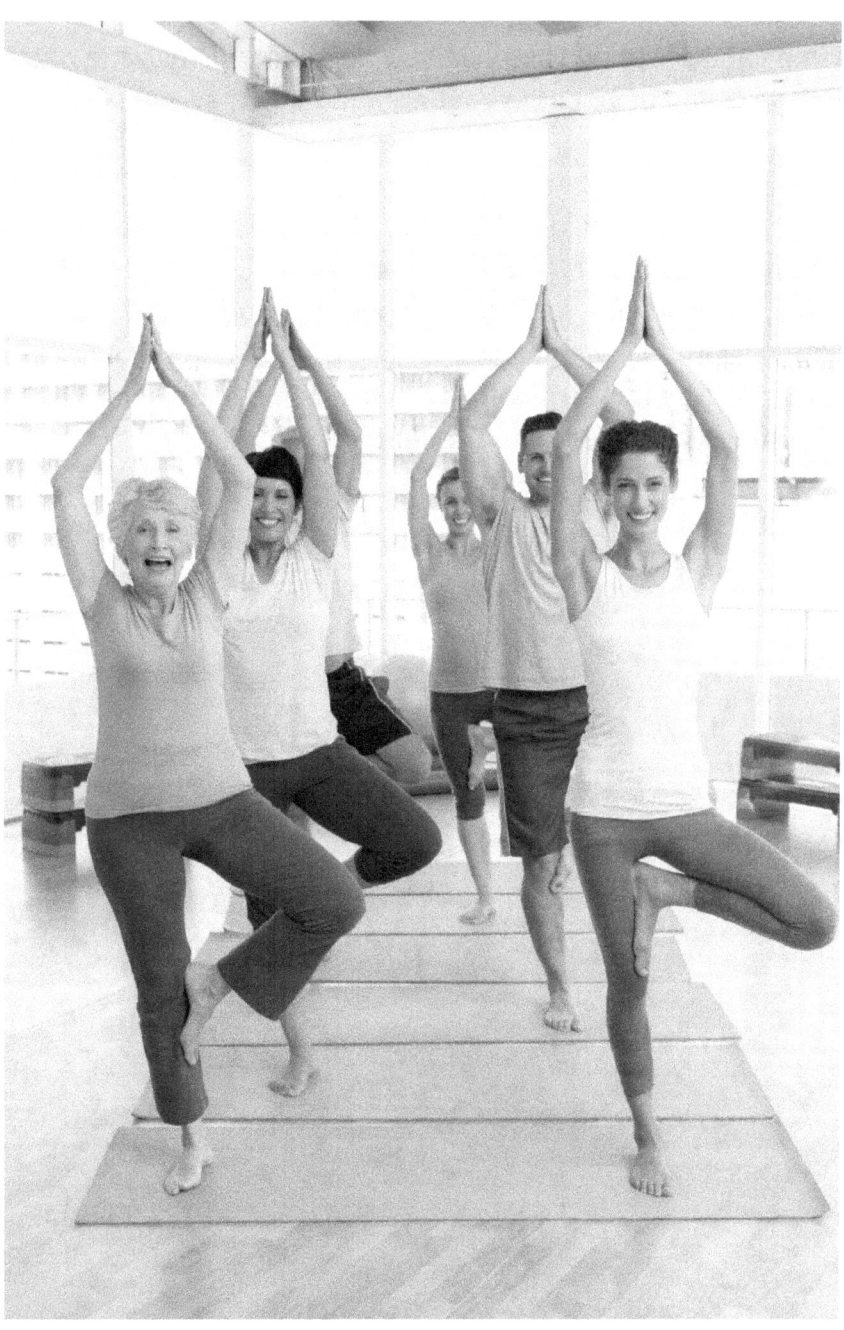

## Instructions
1. Begin standing upright in Mountain Pose.
2. Shift your weight to your right foot.
3. Bend your left knee and lift it upwards as much as you can. You might not be able to get your foot completely off of the ground.
4. Turn your knee outwards so your legs create a figure four. Place your foot flat against your right ankle, calf, or inner thigh. Do not rest your foot against your knee. Activate your core to maintain your balance.
5. Sweep your hands overhead and place your palms together. Leave them here, or bring them down into Prayer Hands against your chest or Reverse Prayer Hands against your back.
6. Hold the pose for a few breaths, and then switch sides.

## Props
1. If you are unable to balance, try this pose next to a chair. Grasp the back of the chair with your right hand while you balance on your right foot, then switch sides.

## Modifications
1. If you're working on the balancing portion, but don't feel completely comfortable, practice this pose near a wall. If you start to fall you can reach out to the wall for support.
2. If balancing is not an option for you, try this pose reclining on the ground. Lie down on your back and create a figure four with your legs by placing the left foot flat against your inner thigh. Let the knee fall outwards, if you can. If this is too intense of a hip and thigh stretch, place the foot against your right ankle. Repeat on the other side.

# Hip Relief

One of the most painful places arthritis takes hold is in the hips. If you have arthritis, you know that you need to exercise those sore or inflamed joints, but in the depths of pain that might just not seem possible. There just aren't very many ways to exercise the hip joints comfortably. That's where yoga comes in.

Yoga offers dozens of poses, from beginner to advanced, that can bring a much-needed stretch and some gentle strengthening to the hips. With yoga, you work at your own pace and listen to your body, helping to deliver the relief you need without making your issues worse.

## Low Lunge

*Sanskrit name: Anjaneyasana*

Low lunge delivers a deep stretch to your hips while building core muscle strength to protect your lower back. This pose is also therapeutic for sciatica pain. It does require you to rest on your knee, so if you have arthritis in your knee you'll have to make modifications (such as using a cushion or towel), or choose to skip this pose. You can try starting with High Lunge instead.

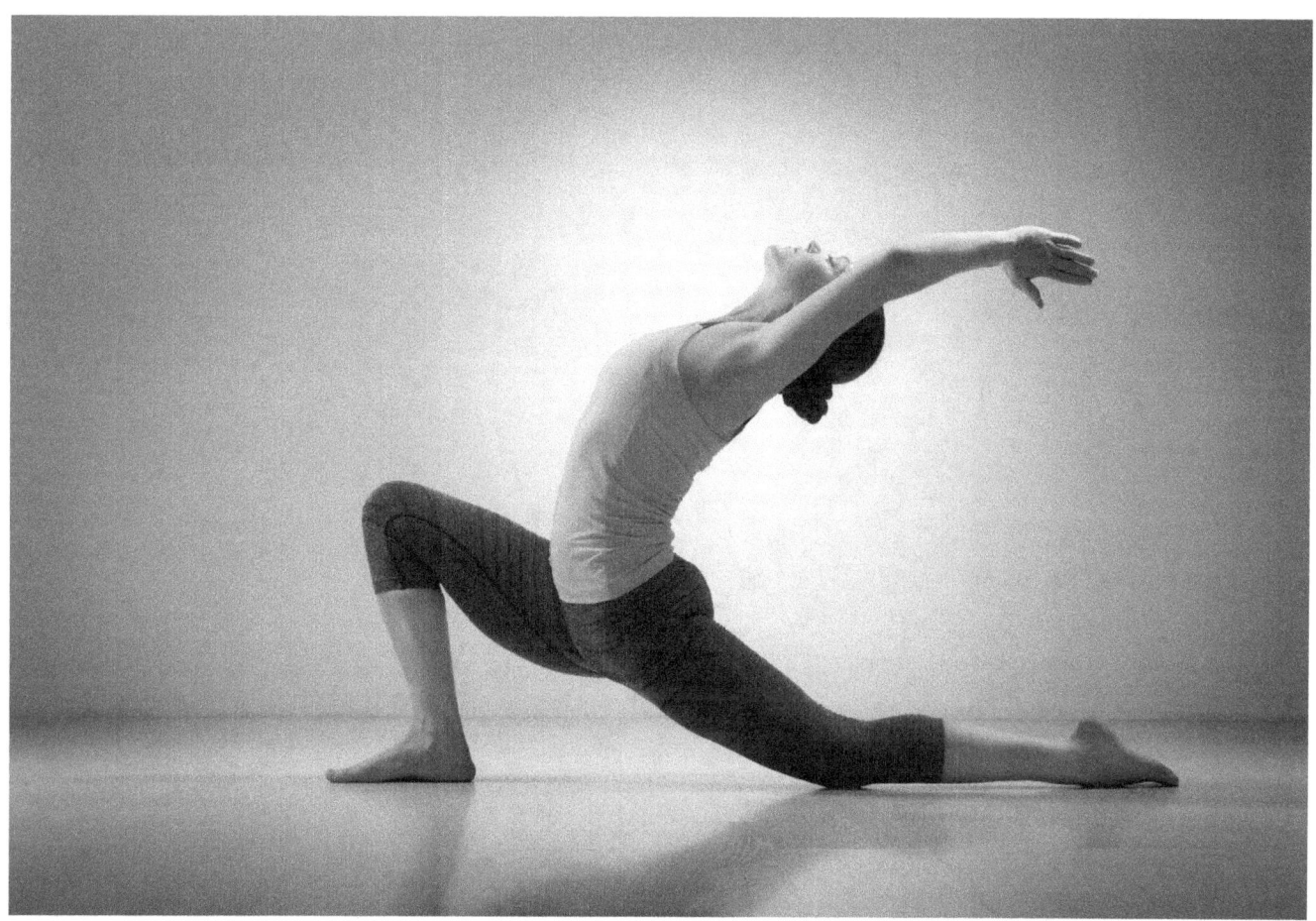

## Instructions
1. Begin in tabletop position. Bring your hands together slightly and move your left foot to the outside of your left hand.
2. Let your hips draw forward and bring your upper body up, lifting your arms above your head with your hands facing inwards towards each other.

## Props
1. If you suffer from sore or inflamed knees, place a blanket or gel pad beneath your knee when in this posture.

## Modifications
1. If you have trouble balancing in this pose at first, use a chair or sturdy nearby object to help support your body.

# High Lunge

***Sanskrit name: Utthita Ashwa Sanchalanasana***

High Lunge is a good alternative to Low Lunge if you're dealing with knee pain. However, it does require more muscular engagement. Eventually, you want to start building up your muscular strength, because a strong and flexible body helps to prevent the injuries that are so common when you're suffering from arthritis and its friend, osteoporosis.

Like Low Lunge, this pose delivers a deep, cleansing stretch to your hips, lengthening your hip flexors while helping to develop core strength. Core strength is likewise important for preventing low back pain and injury. Because this pose stretches out the front of your body, it's also a good tonic for digestive discomforts.

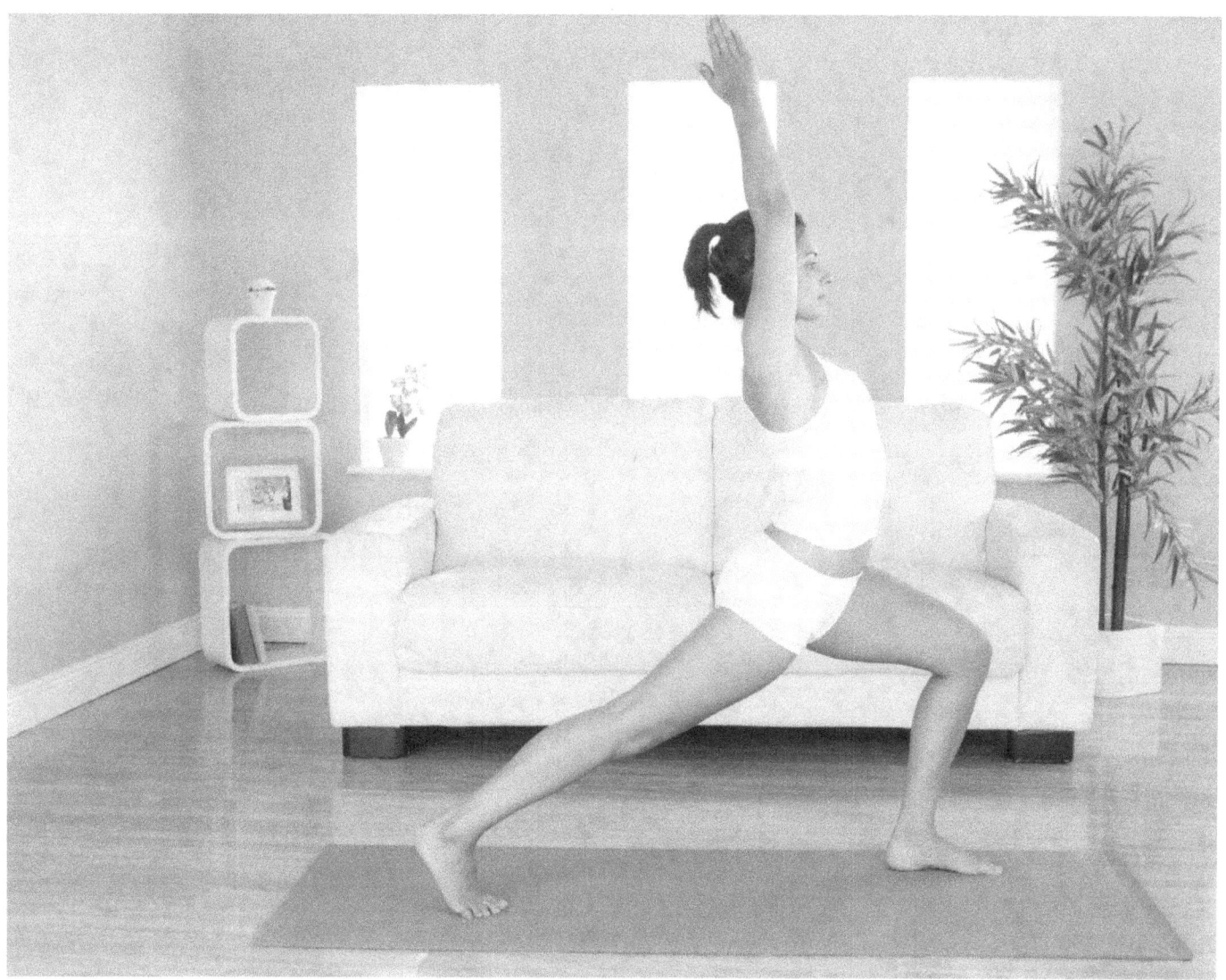

***Instructions***
1. Begin in Standing Forward Fold, palms on the floor. On the inhale, bring your left foot through your hands and step your right foot back, resting on the balls of your right foot. Your left foot should be flat against the earth.
2. Lengthen your torso forward. Rest here with your hands flat against the ground for one breath, and then lift up your torso and sail your arms upwards or rest your hands against your upper thigh.
3. Strengthen your legs to maintain your balance and breathe deeply to open the chest and front body.
4. Take a few breaths in your chosen position, and then switch sides. Transition through Downward Facing Dog if you'd like.

***Modifications***
1. If the balancing aspect of this pose is too much, lower your back knee to the ground. If that is still too much, place both hands on either side of your front foot.
2. You can use a nearby object to help you keep your balance.

# Warrior I Pose

*Sanskrit name: Virabhadrasana I*

Warrior I Pose is a foundational yoga posture that you'll find in most yoga classes. Along with brining a stretch to the hips with the slight lunge, and opening the chest, this pose can also bring relief for sciatica pain. For those who want to get deeper into backbends, the Warrior I pose provides a slight bend to the back that can help you prepare for more intense backbends.

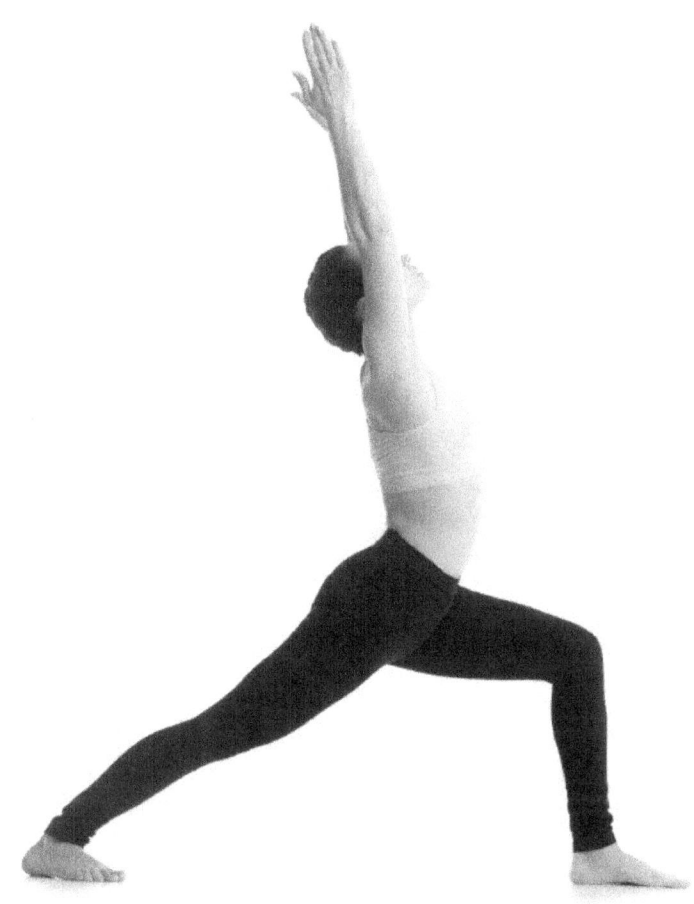

*Instructions*
1. Begin in Mountain Pose.
2. Step your right foot forward about four feet, or as much as is comfortable.
3. Turn your left foot inward at a 45-degree angle, while your right foot faces forward.
4. Attempt to square your pelvis as much as possible with the front of the mat. Bend your right knee to a 90-degree angle. Make sure your knee is not collapsing inwards. You can check this by making sure you can see your right big toe on the inside of your knee when you look down.
5. Lift your arms over your head. Your hands should be facing inwards towards each other.

6. Breathe deeply to open the chest and create a slight backbend. Hold this posture for 30 seconds, or as long as you need.
7. Repeat on the other side.

**Modifications**
1. If you are dealing with arthritis pain in your shoulders, if may not be comfortable to hold your arms over your head. Instead, place your hands on your hips, hold them in Prayer Hands, or get a deep shoulder stretch with Reverse Prayer Hands, if you can.

# Goddess Pose

*Sanskrit name: Utkata Konasana*

Goddess Pose is one of the best ways to open up your hips and bring a delicious but powerful stretch to your hips and inner thighs. Along with the benefits it delivers to your hips, Goddess Pose also opens your chest and strengthens your core. Although this is a restorative pose, enter with caution as the stretch to the hips and thighs can be as powerful as the goddess this pose was named after!

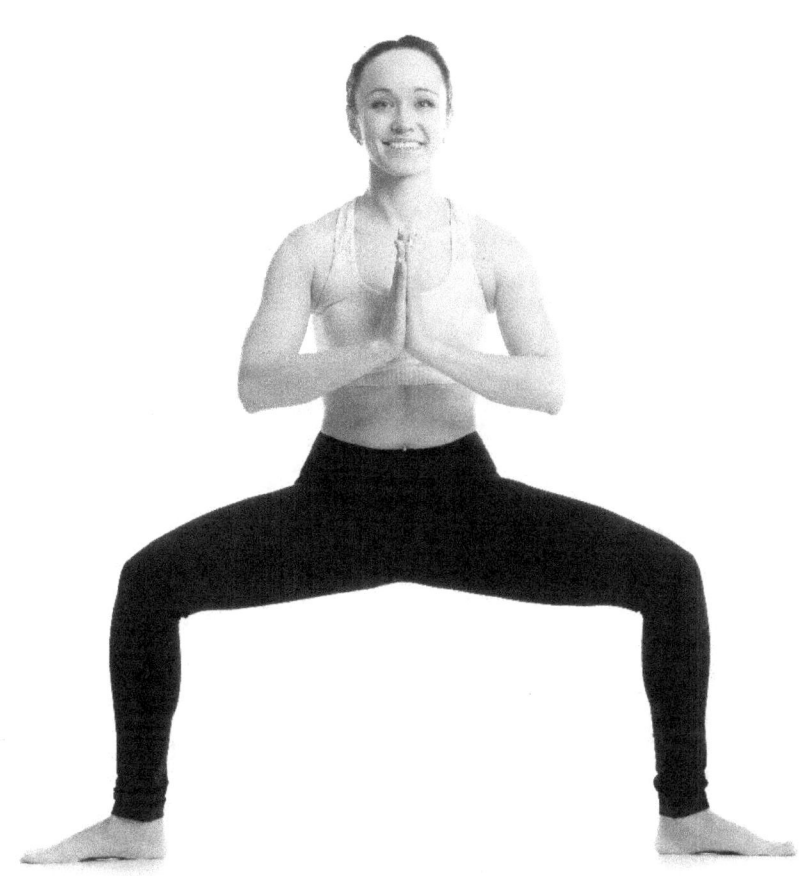

## Instructions
1. Begin standing upright in Mountain Pose.
2. Step your left foot to the back of the mat, then turn both of your feet facing outwards. You should be facing the side of your mat with your legs spread and your toes pointing to the sides.
3. Bend your knees to the degree of your comfort until you feel a stretch in your thighs and hips.
4. Lift your chest and upper body. Ensure that your shoulders are not tense.

5. Lift your arms above your head for a chest opener or slight backbend.
6. Breathe here for as long as is comfortable. You may feel some burning and shaking in your thighs. This is normal; however, you should not feel any sharp pain. If you feel sharp pain, exit the pose gently.

***Modifications***
1. If you have soreness in your shoulders, hold your hands together against your chest in Prayer Hands. If necessary, you can gently place the palms on the knees for balance, but do not hunch.

# Reclining Pigeon Pose

*Sanskrit name: Supta Kapotāsana*

Pigeon Pose brings a very intense stretch to the hips. Although it's a powerful pose, it might not be right for everyone and has been known to put unnecessary strain on shoulders and knees. Instead, try this modification, Reclining Pigeon Pose or Supine Pigeon Pose, for a slightly more gentle take on the yoga classic.

When you're sitting behind a desk or the wheel of a car all day, you also start to shorten your IT band. Your IT band is the connective tissue that runs from your pelvis down the outside of your leg and down your shin. A tight IT band could be causing unnecessary strain on your hip joints. This pose helps to counteract that.

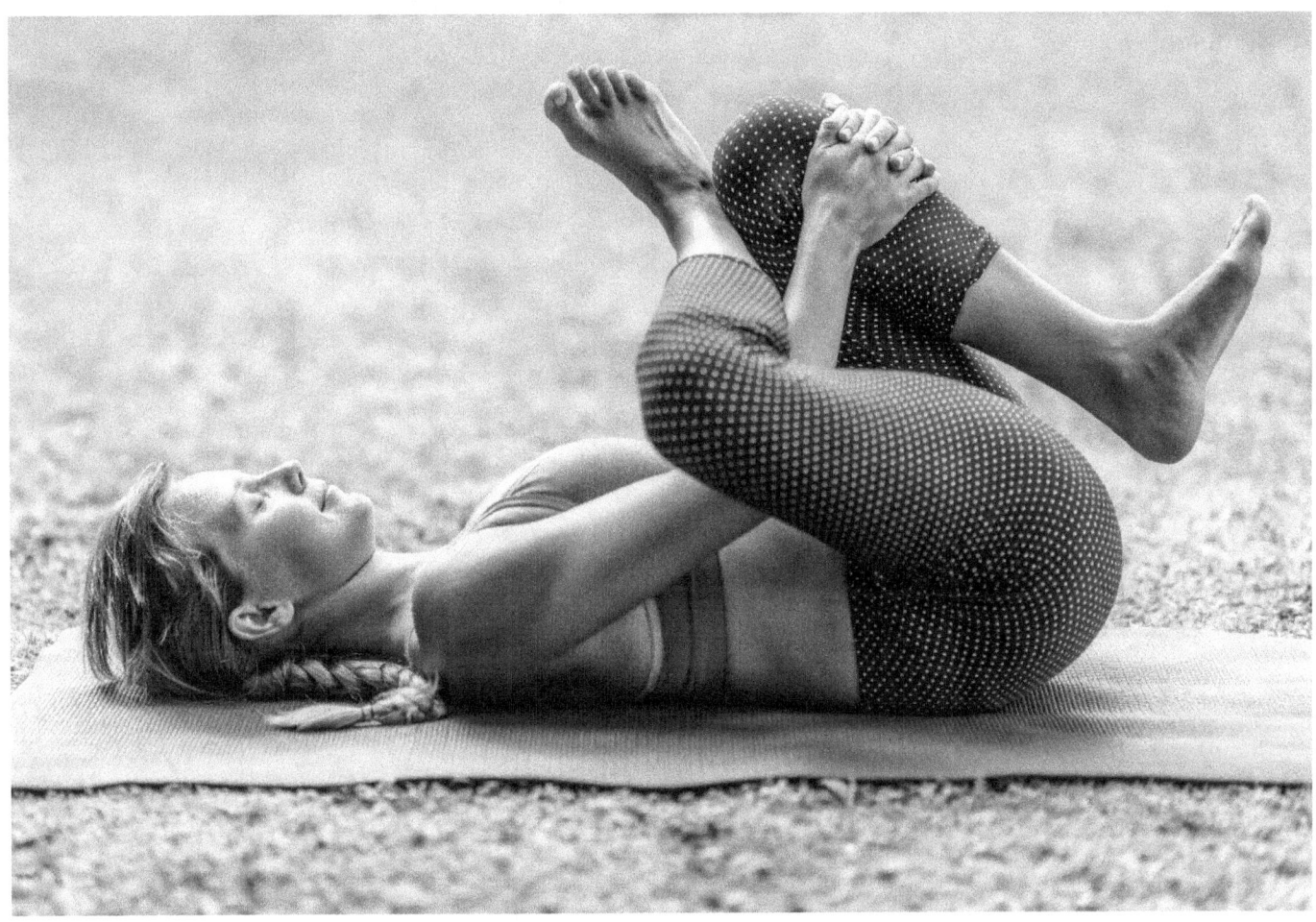

## Instructions
1. Begin on your back with your knees bent.
2. Cross your right ankle over your left thigh. Cross where ever it feels comfortable, as long as you do not rest your right leg against your left knee.
3. Lace your fingers behind your left thigh. If you are able to, lift your left leg towards your face. This will deepen the stretch in your hip. Do not lift or put any strain on your neck.
4. Breathe deeply and hold the pose as long as you need.
5. Repeat on the other side.

## Props
1. If you do not have the flexibility in your shoulders to reach your leg, you can loop a strap around your thigh and hold on to the strap instead as you gently coax your leg closer to your face.

## Modifications
1. If it's time for a deeper stretch, lace your fingers around your shin instead of the back of your thigh.

# Restorative Child's Pose

*Sanskrit name: Salamba Balasana*

Child's Pose is a key yoga posture that everyone should have in their repertoire. Child's Pose is grounding and relaxing, while granting a space-opening stretch to your hips. One of the best things about Child's Pose is that you can control how much of a stretch you want based on how much you spread your hips. It's also an easy pose to modify.

When we add a cushion or support under the upper body, this makes the pose more restorative, so you can spend more time in the pose without causing any strain. Restorative Child's Pose is a perfect gentle stretch to add in at the end of the day, especially when arthritis pain is keeping you up at night. For this pose you'll need a bolster or large pillow.

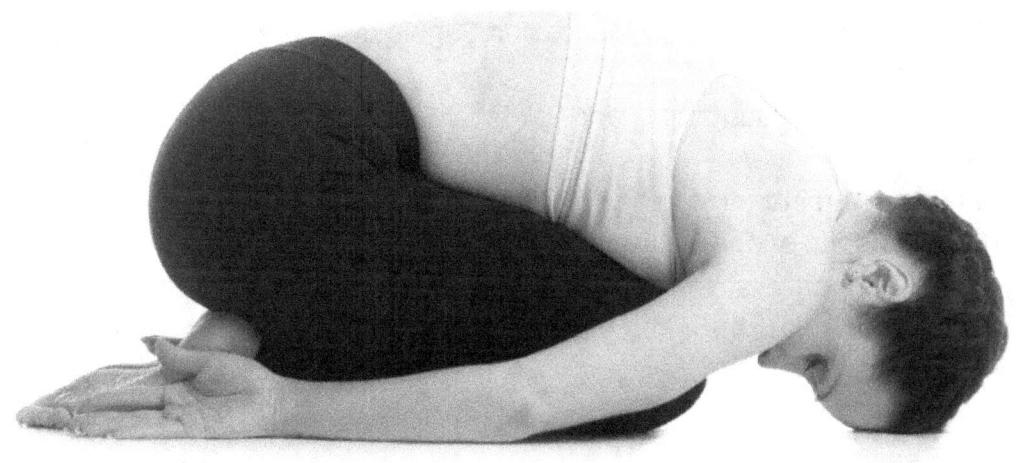

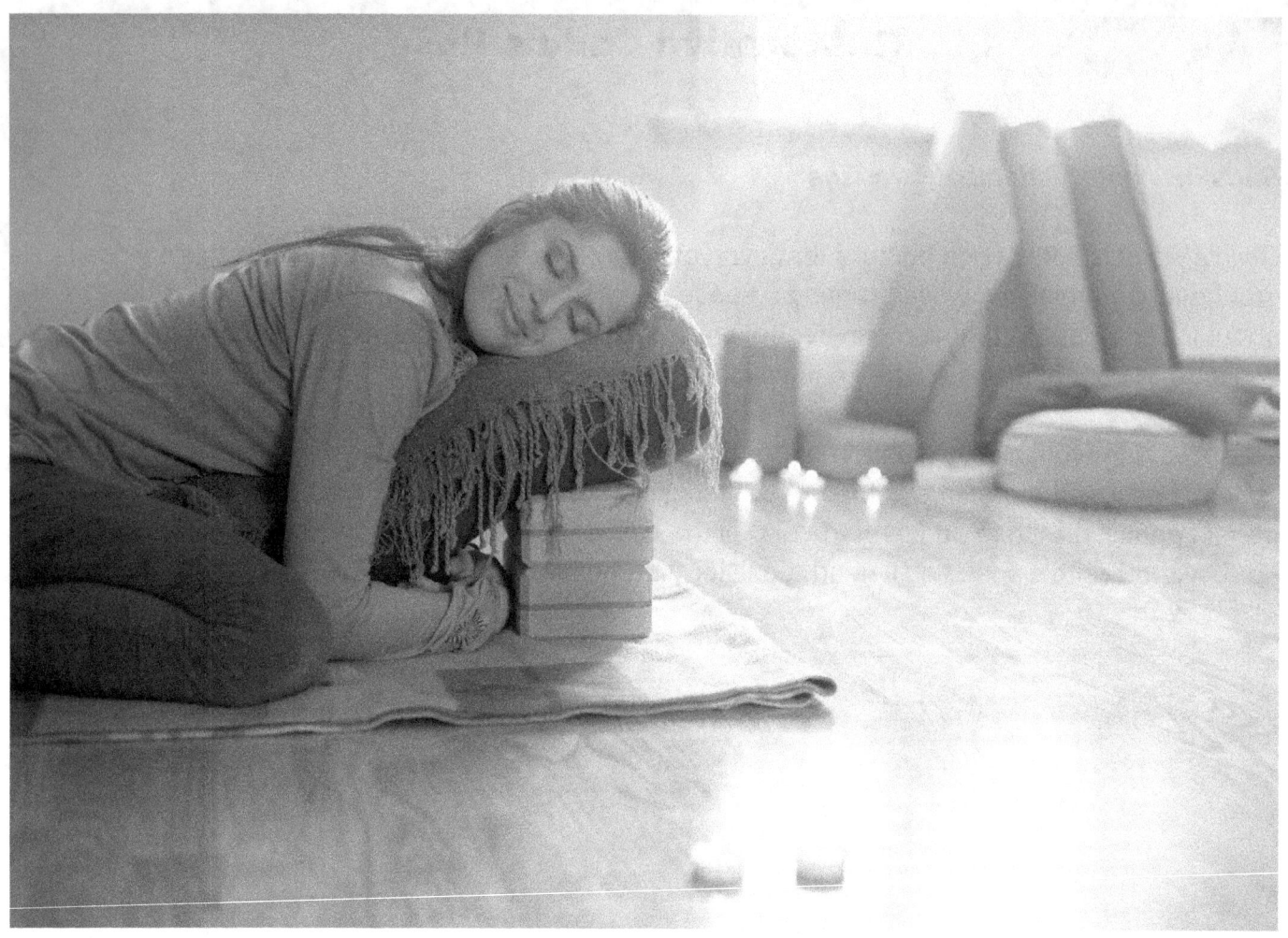

### *Instructions*
1. Sit on your heels with the tops of your feet flat against the earth. Spread your knees outwards to your level of comfort.
2. Drape your body over your thighs, and stretch your arms forward. This would be traditional Child's Pose.
3. To make this pose restorative, place a bolster, large pillow, blocks, or stack of blankets beneath your torso to support your body.
4. You can keep your arms stretched forward, or allow them to rest by your side, whichever is most comfortable. Adjust the width of your knees to your desired stretch.
5. Relax in this pose as long as is needed. Six minutes or more would be appropriate.

### *Props*
1. This pose calls for a bolster, pillow, blocks, or stack of blankets.
2. If you have sore knees, you can also place a blanket beneath them.

# Happy Baby Pose

*Sanskrit name: Ananda Balasana*

This pose is a fantastic restorative hip stretch. It also gently massages your lower back and is deeply calming for the central nervous system. That's why this pose is often performed towards the end of a yoga class, to prepare for Corpse Pose. This is a great pose to add at the end of your practice right before bed.

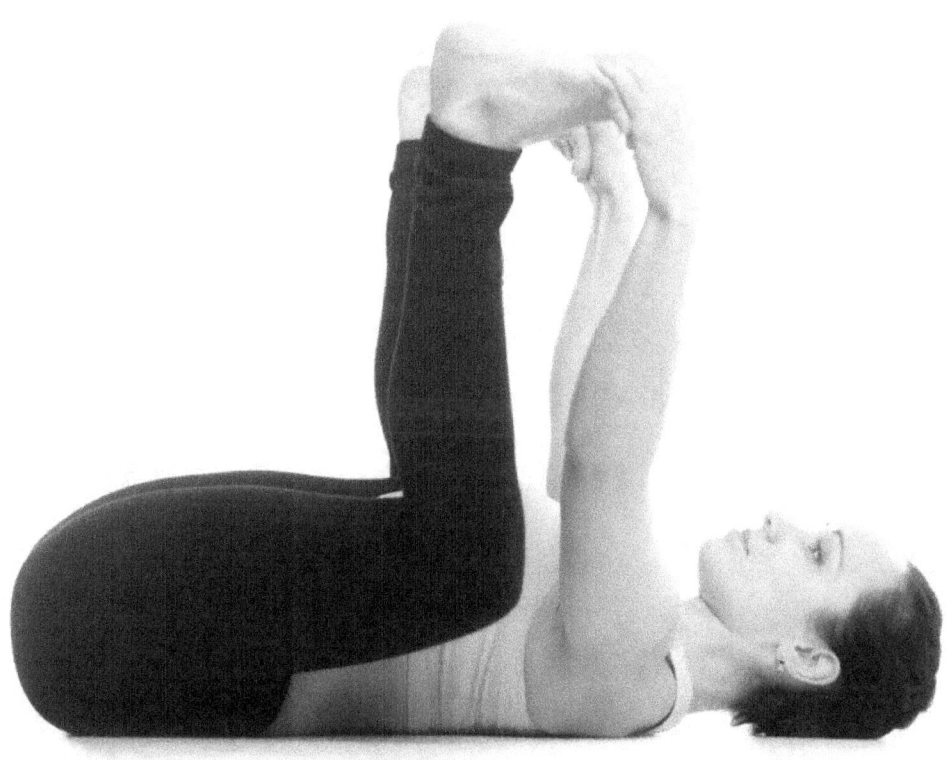

## Instructions
1. Begin by lying on your back on your yoga mat, then bring your knees in towards your chest.
2. Hold on to the outside of your feet and move your knees towards your armpits.
3. Straighten your legs to the best of your ability, just enough to deliver a gentle stretch to your hips and shoulders. Your ankles should be stacked above your knees.
4. If possible, rock back and forth sideways, to give your lower back a stretch and massage.

## Props
1. If you cannot reach your feet, do this pose one leg at a time. Bend one knee towards you and loop a strap around the middle of your foot, then assume the pose with one leg, holding the strap with one hand.

# Fire Log Pose

***Sanskrit name: Agnistambhasana***

This pose is pretty intense for the hips, so you'll want to work your way up to it with more gentle poses, like Child's Pose, first. If you can get to the point where you are doing this pose on a regular basis, you'll practically have new hips. If sciatica pain is also a problem for you, this is one of the best poses for treatment and prevention of that.

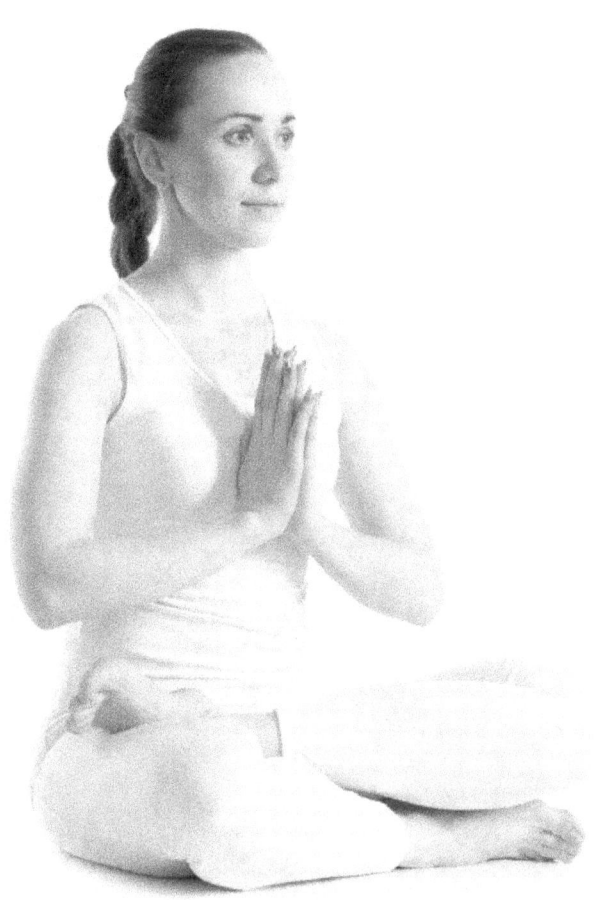

## Instructions
1. Sit on the floor, ideally on a folded blanket, with your knees bent and both feet flat on the floor.
2. Collapse your right leg so the outside of your leg is on the floor and your foot is in front of your pelvis, as if you were sitting crisscross applesauce.
3. Stack your left leg on top of the right, with your left foot resting just below your right knee.

4. Ideally, your legs will lay flush against each other, but realistically, your left knee will probably not reach your right foot. That is perfectly fine, just work on lowering it slowly to the best of your ability.
5. Breathe in this pose for as long as is needed. It is a restorative pose, so you can take your sweet time here, then switch to the other side.

**Modifications**
1. If you'd like to make this pose more intense, straighten your torso, then drape it forward. Inch your hands forward to create length in the spine.

# Lizard Pose

*Sanskrit name: Utthan Pristhasana*

Lizard Pose is an incredibly intense hip stretch, so you don't want to do this pose at the beginning of your practice. Even for experts, this pose is best added in after you've already warmed up the hips and thighs. If you are new to yoga, this is a good pose to have on your radar to work your way up to, but you don't want to try it during your first sessions. However, once you can tackle this pose, it will bring an amazing stretch to the ligaments surrounding your hips.

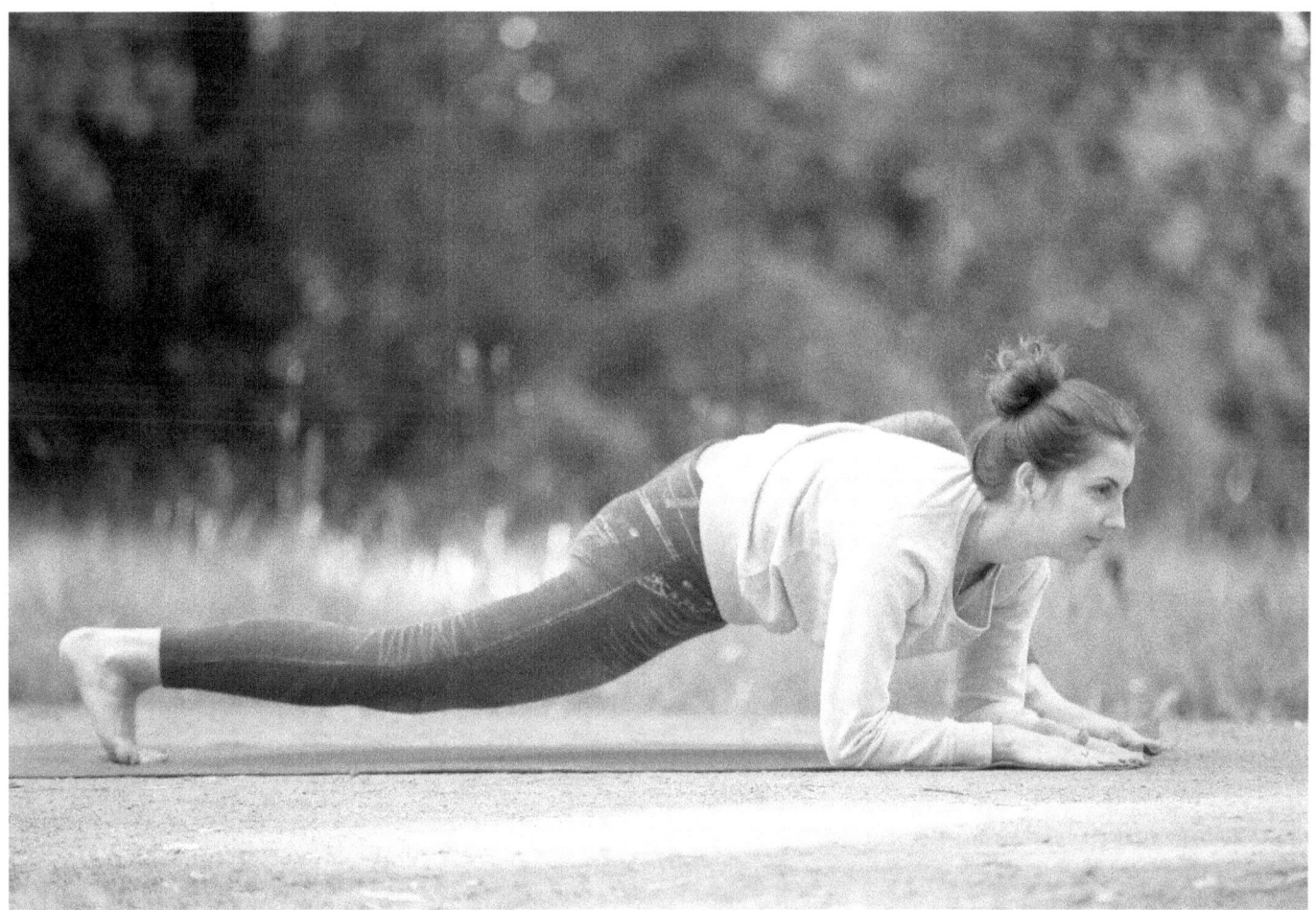

## Instructions
1. Begin in Downward Facing Dog Pose.
2. Lunge your right leg forward to the outside of your right arm and come down to rest your forearms on the earth. Your foot should be parallel with your elbow.
3. Do not collapse your neck and chin. Instead, keep your chest open and chin lifted, parallel with the ground.
4. Keep your back leg lifted to work those leg muscles.
5. Breathe in the pose for as long as possible, then release into Downward Facing Dog.

*Props*
1. If you are not able to reach your forearms to the ground yet, don't worry. Place a block or bolster beneath your arms. You can also stay on your hands.

*Modifications*
1. If you have arthritis in your shoulders, this pose might not be ideal. However, you can try lowering your back knee to remove some of the pressure from your shoulders.

# Knee Pain

If you have arthritis in your knees, your knees are likely very fragile and prone to injury. When practicing yoga, this means you'll have to take extreme care to ensure you don't injure your knees further.

The postures in this chapter are meant to bring a gentle stretch, and sometimes even a challenge to your knees. Implement them into your routine with care. It might even be best to consult a yoga instructor and practice them under his or her supervision first.

When practicing these poses alone, have props like straps and blankets at hand. You should listen to your body and do not push yourself beyond your limits. A burning sensation in your muscles is normal, but any pain – especially a sharp pain – indicates that you should immediately and carefully exit the pose.

You may only be able to comfortably hold these poses for a few seconds and may not be able to enter the full expression of the pose. That's okay! Working your way up to these poses takes practice, but know that each time you mindfully practice one of these poses, you're doing your body a favor.

## Wide Angle Seated Forward Bend

*Sanskrit name: Upavistha Konasana*

This pose provides a much needed stretch to your inner knees, thighs, hips, and ankles. In fact, it's considered one of the best poses for arthritis pain. It's also a deeply relaxing pose, so add this into your routine before bed or after a hard day.

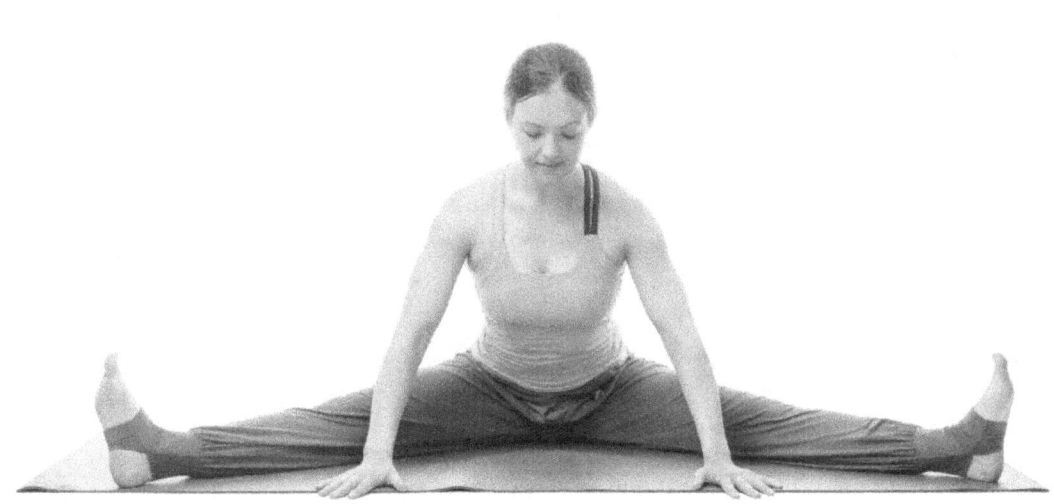

**Instructions**
1. Sit upright on your yoga mat with your legs straight in front of you.
2. Open up your legs as wide as feels comfortable. To give yourself more space, you may sit up on a folded blanket.
3. Press through the heels and activate your thighs.
4. Sit up straight, lengthening through the crown of your head, and then drape your upper body forward between your legs.
5. You may rest on your forearms or inch your arms forward as in Child's Pose.
6. Remain breathing in the pose for as long as is comfortable.

**Props**
1. If you cannot reach your torso to the floor, rest your upper body on a bolster, or support yourself with your palms on the floor.

# Standing Figure Four

*Sanskrit name: Ardha Utkatasana*

Standing Figure Four Pose, also knowns as Half Chair Pose, brings a nice stretch to your outer legs, glutes, lower back, and of course, your knees. The standing version of this posture also builds muscles in the legs and challenges your core. Relieving arthritis pain isn't just about gaining flexibility; it's also about building muscular strength that helps to prevent injury further down the line.

If the standing version of this posture is too intense or challenging, see the instructions below for how to modify the pose to make it more friendly to your needs.

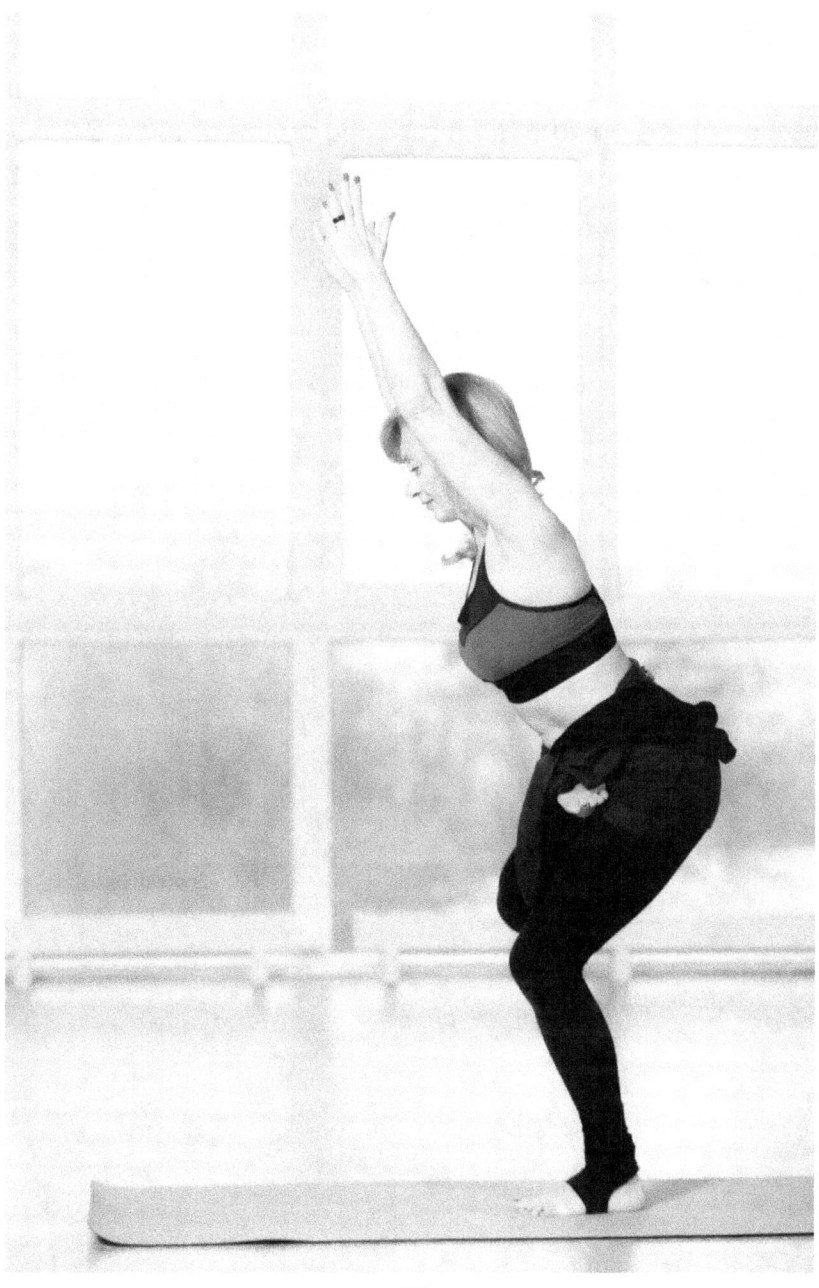

## Instructions
1. Begin standing in Mountain Pose. Bend your right knee slightly.
2. Cross your left leg over your right, with your left ankle resting just above the right knee. Be careful not to cross directly on the knee, as this will put too much pressure on the joint.
3. Bend your right knee as much as is comfortable, until you feel a stretch.
4. Bring the arms upward with palms facing toward the body. You can also hold your hands against your chest in Prayer Hands.
5. Breathe in the pose as long as needed. Repeat on the other side.

## Props
1. If you have trouble maintaining your balance, practice this pose behind a chair. Hold onto the chair for balance instead.

## Modifications
1. If you are having trouble balancing, but would like to deepen the stretch, fold over your bent leg and place your hands on the ground, bending your right leg as much as needed to reach the ground. If reaching the ground is not possible, place your hands on a block.
2. For a milder version of this posture, try it reclining on the ground. Bend your knees so your feet are flat on the mat, then cross your left ankle over your right leg to create a figure four.

# Warrior II Pose

*Sanskrit name: Virabhadrasana II*

Warrior II Pose is a foundation pose in the yoga canon. Most yoga classes will include this pose, so it's good to master it on your own. This pose delivers strength building to the legs and arms, while broadening across the chest, and bringing a gentle stretch to the knees and thighs. Because this is a more engaged pose, you must exercise caution when practicing and be sure to not overwork your knees.

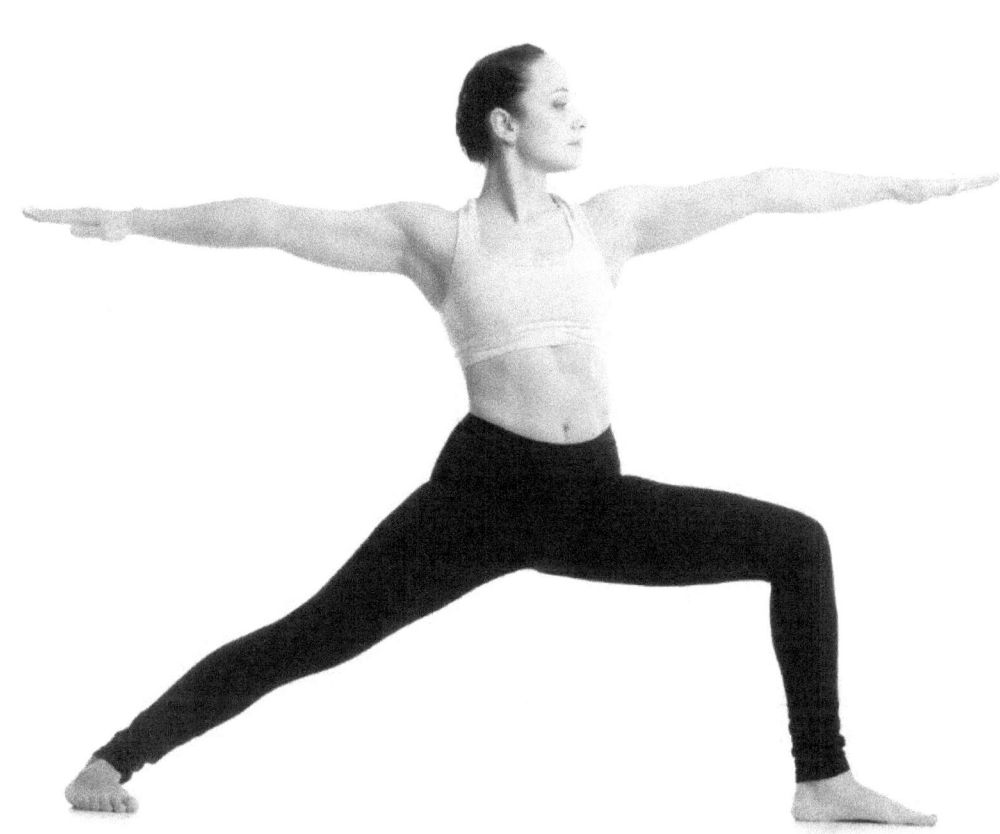

### Instructions
1. Begin standing in Mountain Pose.
2. Step your right leg backwards on the mat about 3–4 feet, depending on your flexibility.
3. Turn your right foot out at a 90-degree angle, but keep your left foot pointed straight ahead. Make sure your heels are in line with each other.
4. Begin to bend the left leg until it is bent at the knee at a 90 degree angle.
5. Stretch your arms out to your sides so they are parallel with the floor.
6. Inhale to broaden across the chest and open your shoulders. Check to make sure your shoulders are not tensing up and moving upwards towards your ears.

7. Activate your core and elongate your tailbone towards the earth.
8. Make sure your front leg is not collapsing inwards. If it is, this can cause pain or even injury in the knee. You should be able to see your big toe through the inside of your knee if you gaze downwards.
9. Turn your neck to the left to gaze over your fingertips.

**Modifications**
1. If you have a sore neck, look straight ahead. Do not turn your neck to look over your hand.
2. If you have sore shoulders, skip the arm posture. Instead place your hands on your hips or anywhere else that is comfortable for you.

# Modified Bound Angle Pose

*Sanskrit name: Baddha Konasana*

Bound Angle Pose is a simple pose that brings a delicious stretch to the inner thighs, hips, and the knees. Unfortunately, the traditional version can be a little too much for some people's fragile knees. This modified version maintains the simplicity and stretching of the original while taking pressure off of the knees and hips.

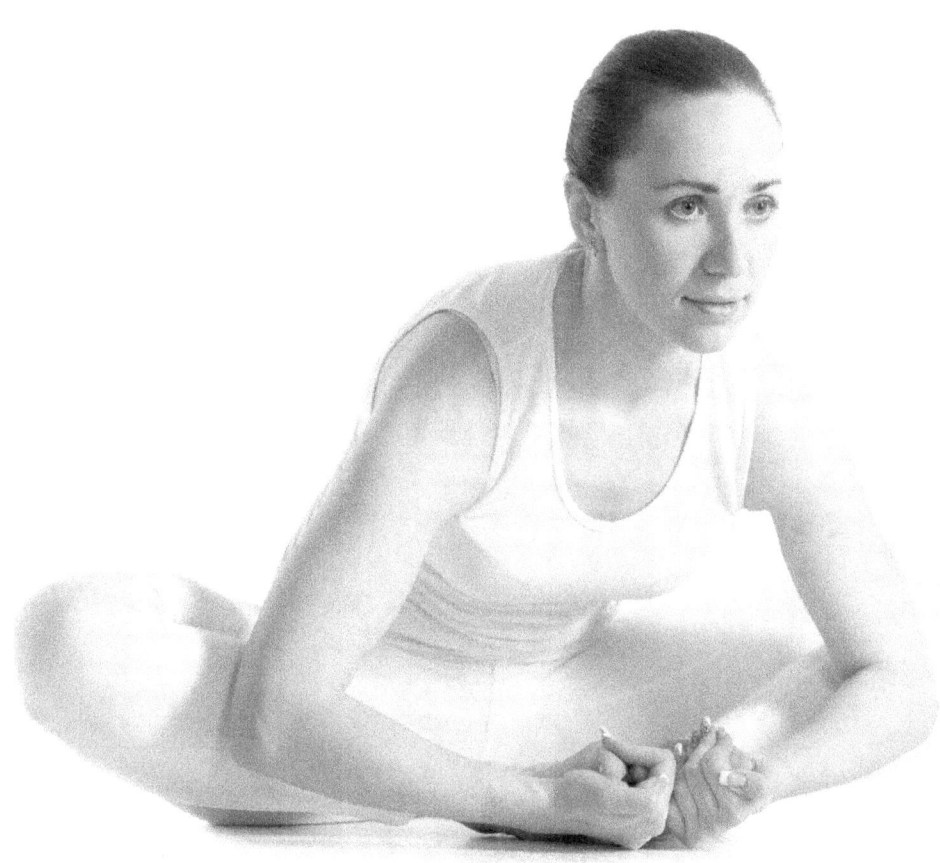

### Instructions
1. Sit upright on your mat with your legs straight in front of you.
2. Bring your feet together so the soles touch and your ankles are resting on the ground. Then bring your feet as close to your pelvis as you can comfortably handle.
3. Place rolled blankets beneath the knees to bring some of the pressure off the joints. Lean forward from the hips if that feels good.
4. Breathe deeply to open the chest and remain in this pose as long as is comfortable.

### Props
1. If resting on the ankles brings pain, place a towel or blanket beneath the ankles.

# Modified Garland Pose

*Sanskrit name: Malasana*

Garland Pose brings a powerful stretch to your legs while opening up your hips. Not many exercises or poses target your ankles, which means our ankles can get pretty tight. Garland Pose is an exception, bringing a stretch to both ankles.

Garland Pose is also a relaxing pose that can help you to see big changes in your hips and lower body. However, it's not really ideal for those with knee pain. This modified version takes your knees into account, delivering a posture that can be done by those with sore and arthritic knees.

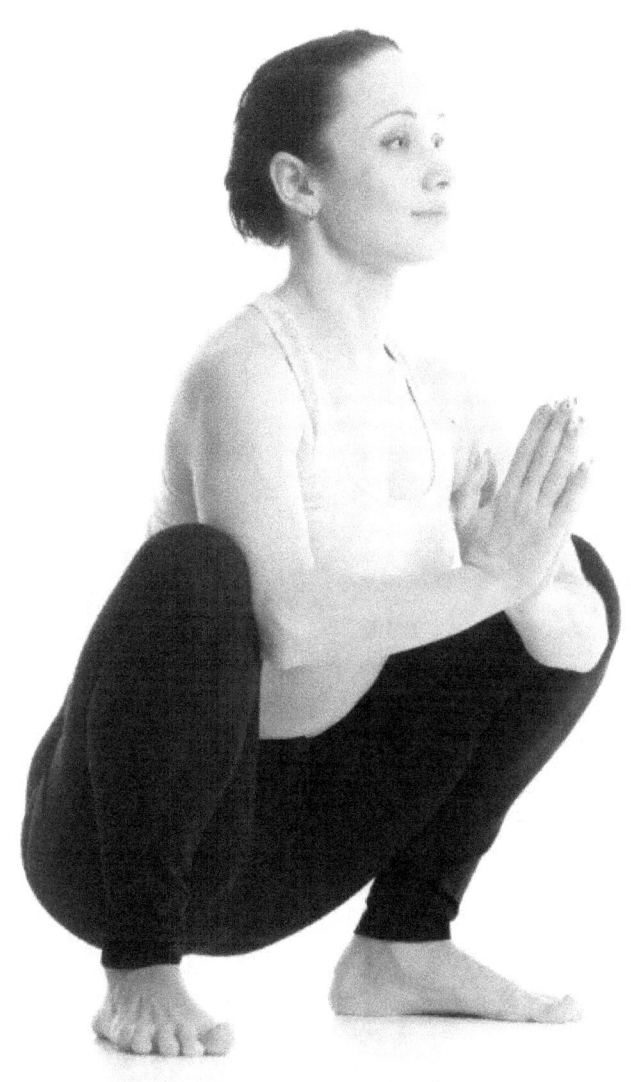

***Instructions***
1. Begin standing upright in Mountain Pose, then squat down. Your heels should touch the ground, but this isn't possible for everybody.
2. If your heels do not touch the ground, place a folded blanket beneath them.
3. To prevent knee pain, place a rolled-up blanket or a cushion behind your knees. Your bent legs will hold the blanket in place.
4. Bring your hands together in prayer pose with your elbows extended wide.
5. Use your elbows to spread your knees outwards and open your hips even more.
6. Breathe here for as long as it is comfortable.

***Modifications***
1. If the balancing aspect of this pose is too much, practice against the wall.

# Extended Triangle Pose

*Sanskrit name: Utthita Trikonasana*

When it comes to poses that open up the entire body, Extended Triangle Pose might just take the cake. It's especially popular with pregnant women. This pose opens up your legs, hips, and lower back, while providing a gentle stretch to the knees and ankles, two areas that are so often neglected. It also opens up the chest and stretches the stomach, bringing relief for digestive discomfort.

Few practices are complete without this pose, although it can be challenging for some who don't have a lot of flexibility in their legs and shoulders. Below, some suggestions for modifications and props will be included to make this pose more accessible for those with arthritis.

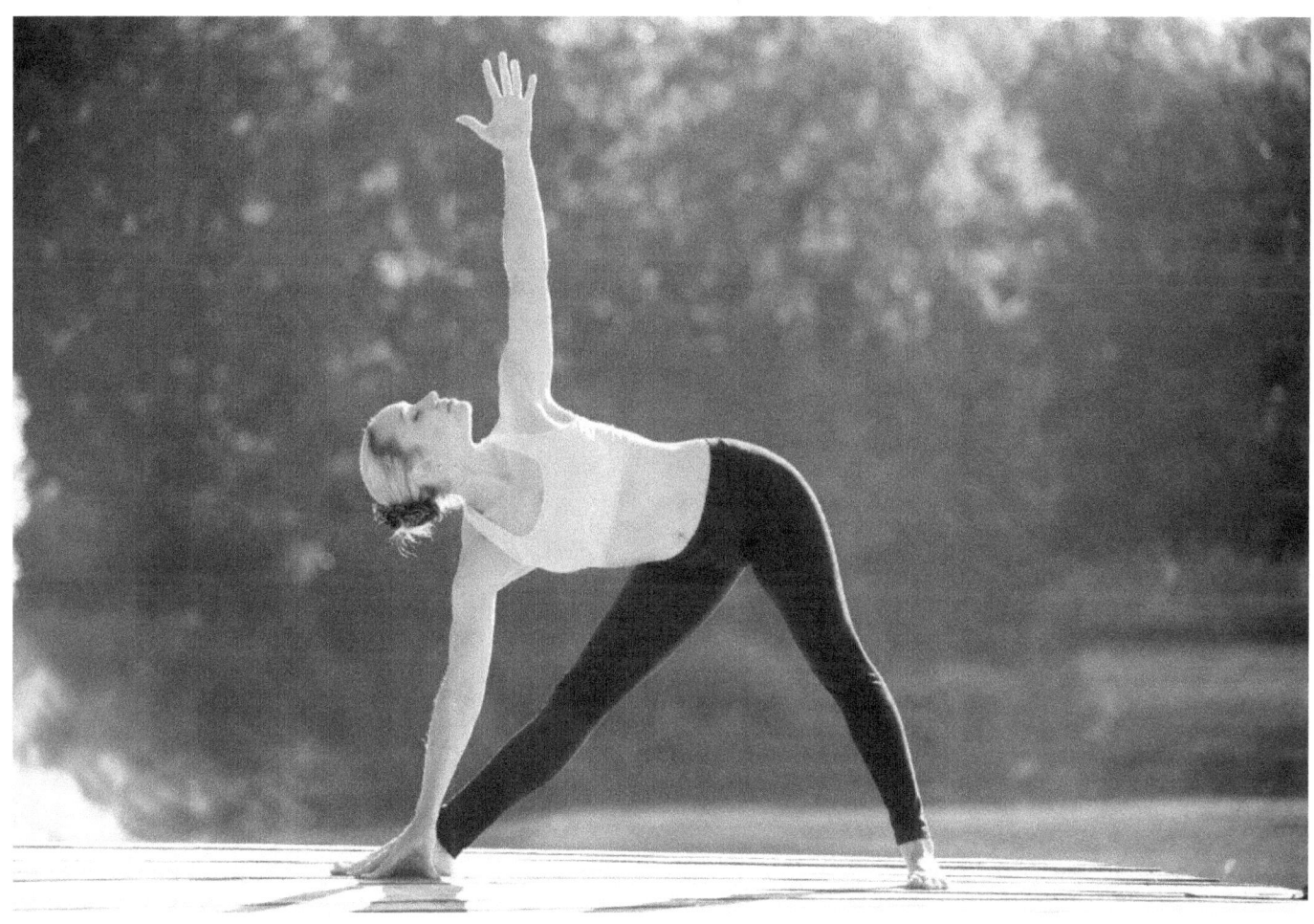

## Instructions

1. Begin in Mountain Pose.
2. From the standing position, step your right foot back 3–4 feet depending on how tight your hips are.
3. Keep your left toes facing forward and turn your right foot out at a 90-degree angle. Make sure your heels are in line with each other.
4. Raise your arms out to either side, palms facing down. Take a deep breath to open up the chest and stretch your arms out even wider.
5. As you exhale, lead with the crown of your head to stretch your body over your left leg as much as possible, keeping your torso parallel with the floor.
6. Place your left hand on the earth to the outside of your left foot, on your shin, or on your thigh, depending on how much flexibility you have in your legs and back.
7. Lift your right arm over your head, stretching upwards to create space in your shoulders.
8. Turn your neck to look upwards towards your hand.
9. Remain in this pose as long as needed, being mindful not to hyperextend your knee.
10. Repeat on the other side.

## Props

1. If you are not able to reach the floor, place your hand on a block instead.

## Modifications

1. For those with neck pain, do not turn your neck to look upwards when in this pose. You should also focus your gaze on one point or close your eyes to avoid straining your neck.

# Modified Easy Pose

*Sanskrit name: Sukhasana*

Easy Pose is a seated posture that helps you to prepare for the more intense pose, Lotus Pose. Easy Pose actually isn't that easy, but it does help to develop the strength needed in the lower back to prevent pain and injury, correct posture, and bring a gentle stretch to the knees. This modification helps to create more space in the lower back for a less strenuous option.

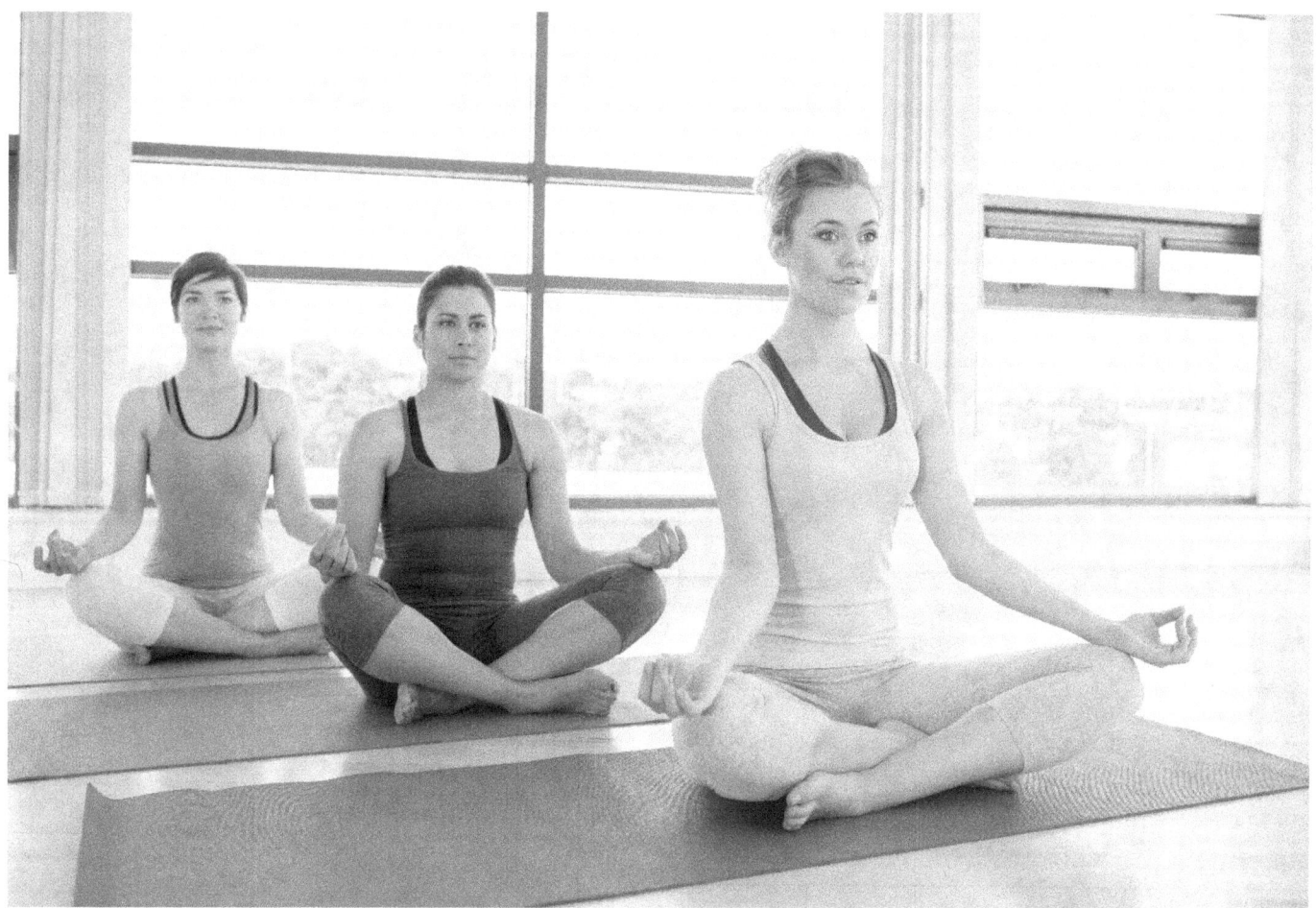

**Instructions**
1. Place a few folded blankets or a block beneath your sitting bones, and inch your buttocks close to the edge of the blanket. Extend your legs in front of you. Make sure your pelvis is in a neutral position.
2. Bring your feet in close to your pelvis and cross your legs at the shins, resting the upper shin against the opposite foot.
3. Sit up straight, reaching the crown of your head towards the sky.
4. Breathe in this position for as long as is comfortable, then switch so the other leg is in front, and continue breathing.

# Half Moon Pose

*Sanskrit name: Ardha Chandrasana*

Half Moon Pose is another standing pose that brings a much-needed stretch to the knees and ankles. It also challenges you to balance, helping to develop core strength to prevent lower back pain and injury. This pose actually opens up the entire body, especially the chest, shoulders, and upper back, so it can be a great tonic after a long day at work.

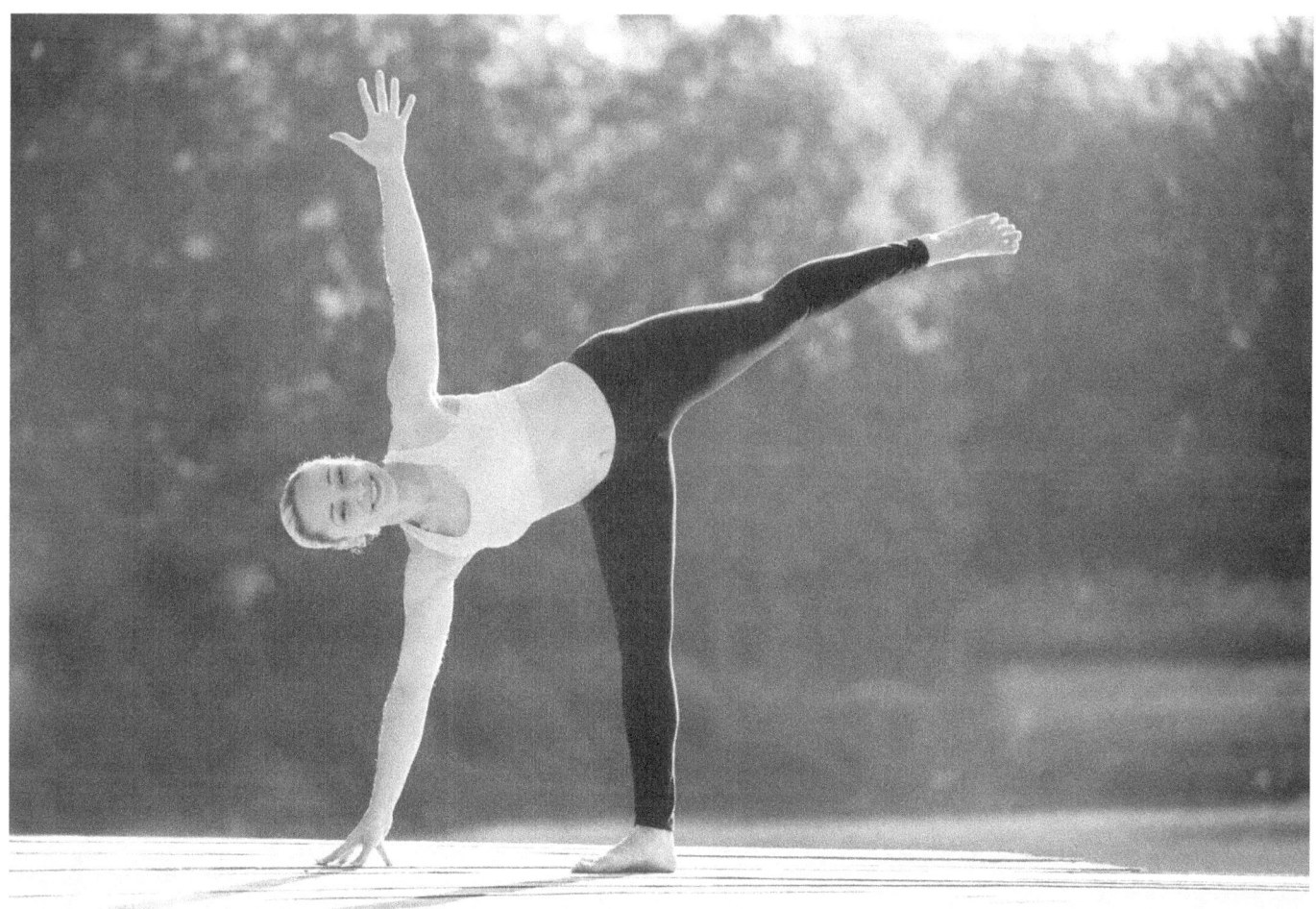

## Instructions
1. Begin in a forward fold.
2. Lift your left leg as far as you can off of the mat.
3. Turn your entire body to the left, rotating your chest open.
4. With one hand flat on the ground, lift your left arm towards the sky.
5. Do not hyperextend your standing knee.
6. Breathe in this pose as long as is comfortable, then repeat on the other side.

## Props
1. If you are not able to reach the floor, place your hand on a block instead.
2. If it is too much strain to lift your arm to the ceiling, place it on your hip and rotate your chest open.

## Modifications
1. For those with neck pain, do not turn your neck to look upwards when in this pose. You should also focus your gaze on one point or close your eyes to avoid straining your neck.
2. If the balancing aspect of this pose is too demanding, practice against a wall.

# Supported Reclining Hero Pose

*Sanskrit name: Supta Virasana*

Hero Pose can be a little intense and uncomfortable. Making it a reclining pose helps to add a restorative element. That said, the reclining position also delivers a more intense (but sustainable) stretch to the thighs and ankles.

Both versions of this pose bring a stretch to the knees. It can be too intense for some, so listen to your body and work at your own pace. You probably shouldn't try this pose right away if you feel like a beginner.

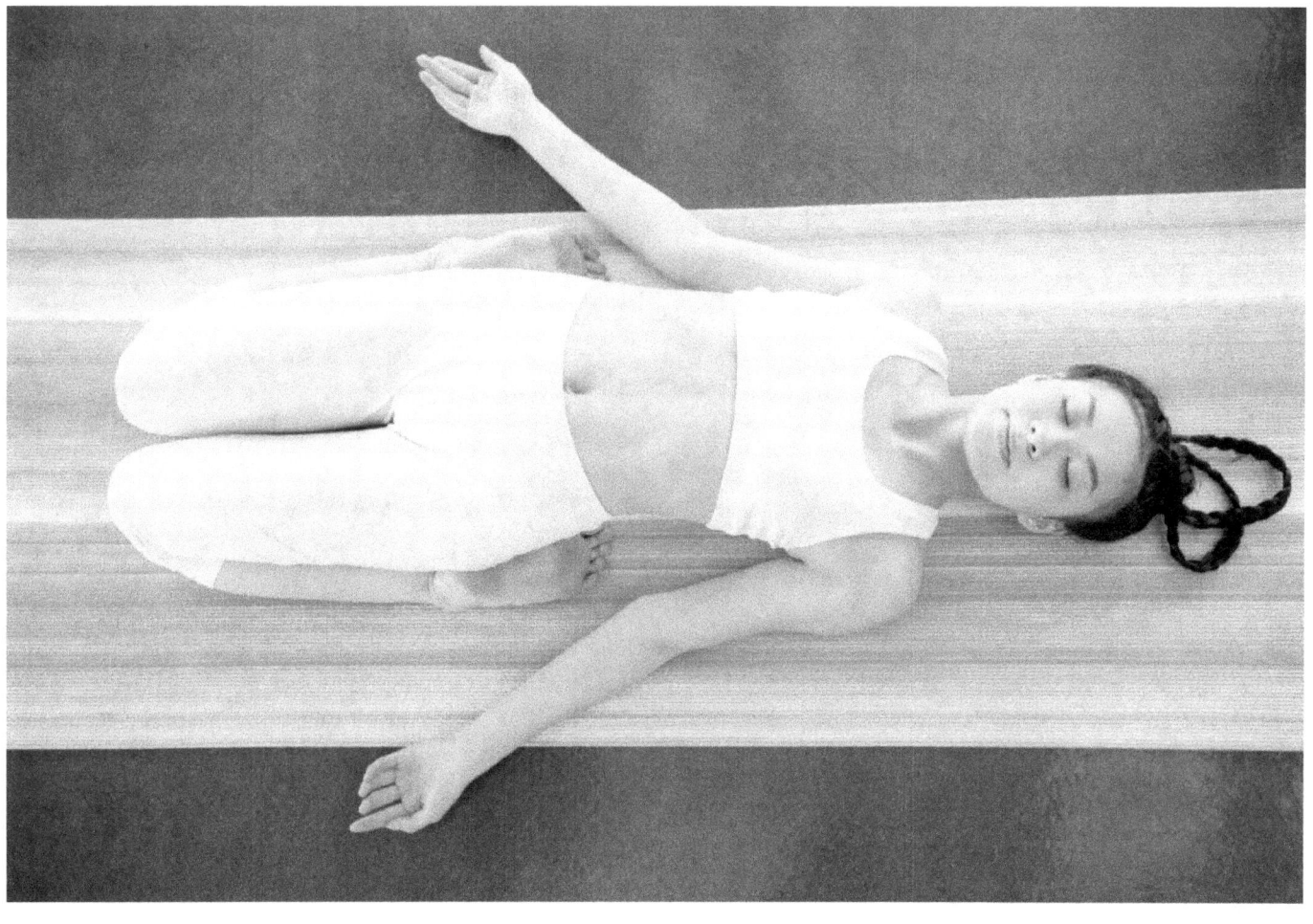

## Instructions
1. Sit on the ground with your knees bent behind you and your feet to either side of your buttocks.
2. Place a large bolster behind your lower back and a pillow to support your head.
3. Lean back to your degree of comfort.

4. You may need to add folded blankets to the bolster until you are reclining at a level that is comfortable for you.
5. Breathe in the pose as long as you like, remaining mindful of the sensations in your knees. If you feel any sharp pains, disengage from the pose immediately.

***Props***
1. If resting on your knees is too painful, try placing a folded blanket beneath them.
2. If the stretch in your knees is too intense, you may also sit on a block.

# Lotus Pose

***Sanskrit name: Padmāsana***

Lotus Pose is one of the most famous poses in yoga, especially for meditation. For those with knee troubles, Lotus Pose can bring a lot of healing or a lot of pain, so it should be practiced with caution. It is certainly not a pose for beginners, so you should work your way up it. The first time you try this pose, you should do so under the supervision of a teacher.

However, if you are able to master this pose, you'll be treated to a wonderful stretch in the hips and knees, while building strength in the lower back that helps to prevent injury and pain.

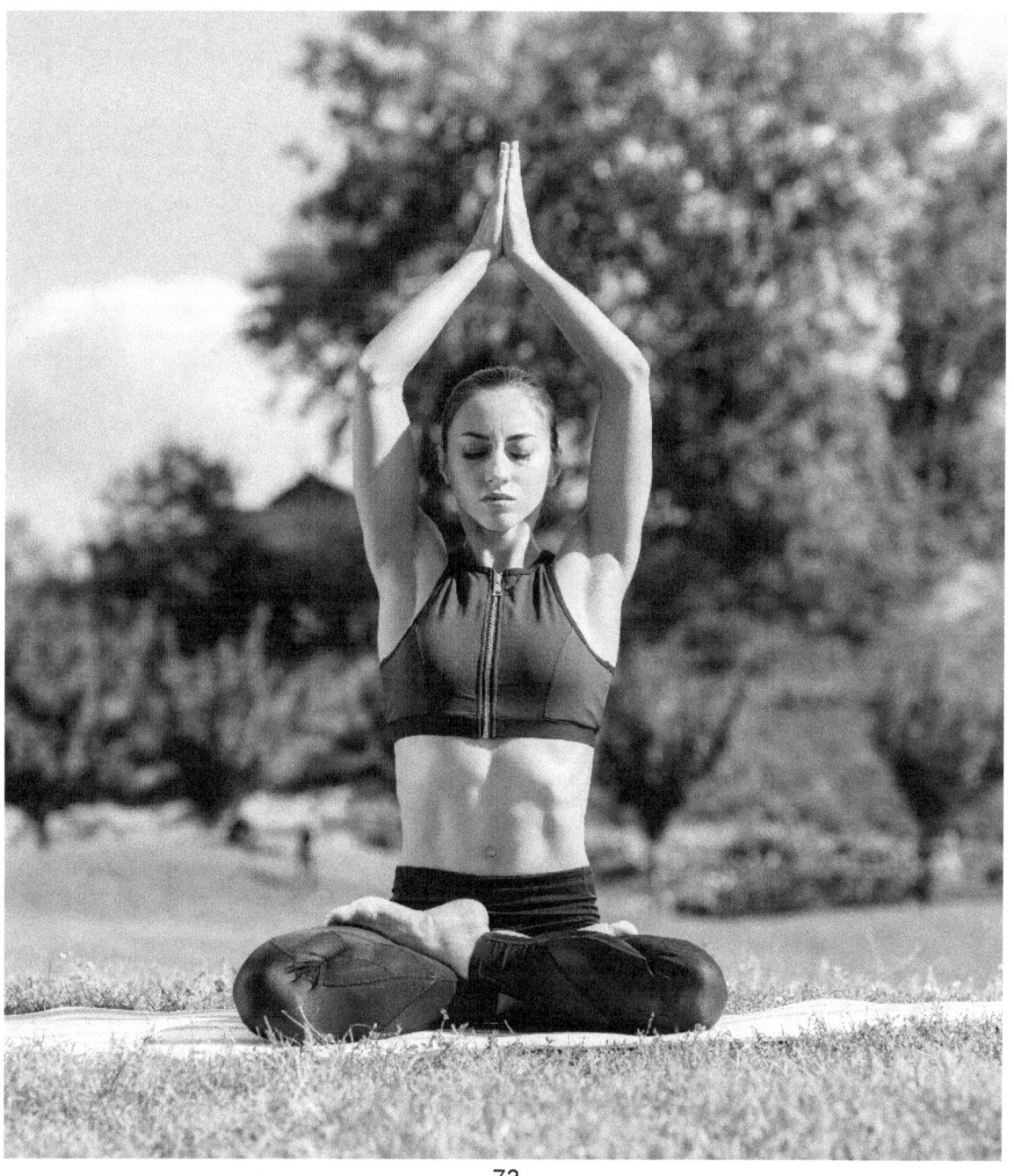

## Instructions
1. After carefully stretching your hips and knees, sit on your yoga mat with your legs in front of you.
2. Bring your right shin and foot into a cradle in your arms.
3. Lodge the right foot into the crease of your left hip.
4. Repeat with the other side so the left leg is crossed in front of the right and both feet are snuggling into the opposite hip.
5. If you are a beginner, only hold the pose for a few seconds before releasing.

## Props
1. If one of your legs does not reach the floor in this pose, support that leg with a folded blanket.

# Releasing the Neck

Most of us spend the day looking down at our phone or computer, sitting behind a desk, and slouching behind the wheel of a car. Because of this sedentary lifestyle we live, we tend to hold a lot of tension and pain in the neck. Since the neck is connected to everything else, tension in the neck can exacerbate arthritis pain in the shoulders and back. It can also cause debilitating headaches.

Those with arthritis pain in the neck know that this is one of the most painful places to have arthritis. When arthritis flares up in the neck, it gets in the way of living your life. Suddenly, you can't drive a car or even read a book without pain. These poses and exercises are gentle enough to bring a stretch to your neck when you are in pain, while helping to release tension and increase mobility.

## Downward Facing Dog

*Sanskrit name: Adho Mukha Svanasana*

Downward Facing Dog is one of the most classic poses in the yoga canon. No yoga practice is complete without Down Dog. This pose delivers a full body stretch from your ankles to your neck. Dangling your neck between your hands allows the weight of your head to gently stretch and open up your neck.

If you have arthritis in your wrists or shoulders this pose may not be ideal. However, if you can work your way up to it, Down Dog can help to build muscles in the shoulders.

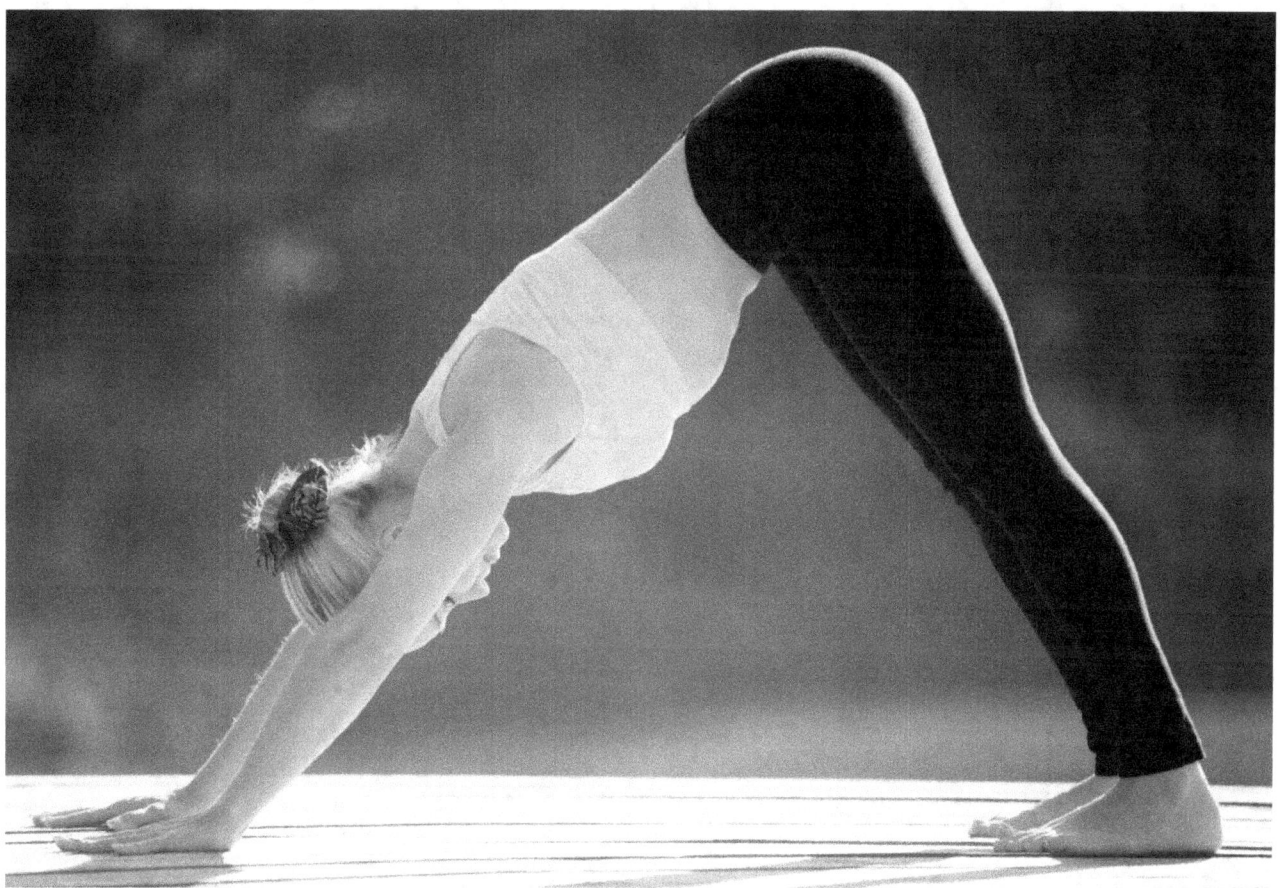

## Instructions

1. Begin on your hands and knees in Tabletop Pose.
2. From there, tuck your toes and lift your hips into the air until your legs are as straight as you can comfortably get them. Those with very flexible ankles will be able to reach their feet to the floor, but most people will be on the balls of their feet.
3. Lengthen your tailbone towards the ceiling, spread your fingers wide, and move your shoulders down your back to create space for the neck to relax. Broaden your chest to create a stretch in the chest and upper back.
4. Breathe in this pose for as long as is comfortable.

## Props

1. If your arms keep splaying outwards, this can put undue pressure on the shoulders. Loop a strap around your arms and pull it tight to keep your arms in alignment. You can press slightly against the strap to open the chest.

## Modifications

1. If your wrist pain is too much to do this pose, try Dolphin Pose instead for a similar stretch.
2. To deepen the pose, alternate between bending your knees and drawing your right and left heel closer to the ground. This will deliver a deeper stretch to the calves.

# Wide Legged Standing Forward Bend

*Sanskrit name: Prasarita Padottanasana*

Prasarita, as it is usually called, delivers the same benefits of a forward fold, but the wide-legged stance allows for a deeper stretch in the inner thigh. It also brings to the table the same calming benefits of inversion poses, but with none of the added tension to the neck, making this a great choice for those with neck pain.

On the topic of neck pain, this is a pose that allows the head to dangle freely, gently elongating and stretching the neck.

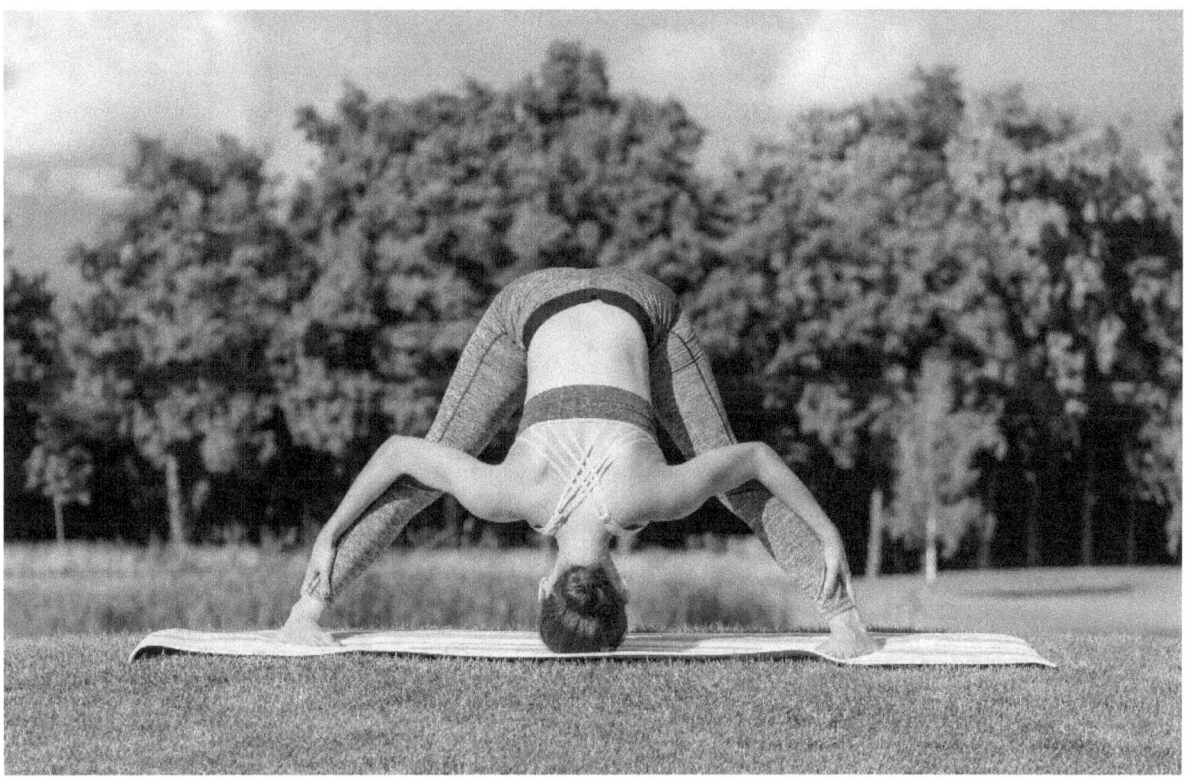

## Instructions
1. Begin in Mountain Pose, then step one leg back about 3–4 feet.
2. Turn both feet so they are facing the same direction.
3. Fold forward until the crown of your head touches the earth, or as far as is comfortable.
4. You can keep your hands on your hips, reach them to the floor, or add in an arm posture for additional benefits.
5. Breathe in the pose as long as is comfortable.

## Props
1. Many people are not able to reach their hands to the floor. In this case, you may place your hands on a block instead until you eventually work your way down to the floor.

## Modifications
1. To deepen the shoulder stretch, add in a Hand Clasp or Reverse Prayer Hands.

# Modified Fish Pose

*Sanskrit name: Matsyasana*

Fish Pose is an intense back bend that really opens up the throat and neck. It might be a little too intense for beginners and those suffering from neck pain, so this modified version is a better option. This pose is amazingly relaxing, so add it towards the end of your practice or before bed. The front body stretch also provides fantastic relief for backaches, tight hips, digestive issues, and respiratory issues. If you also are struggling with autoimmune disease, that powerful combination makes this an ideal pose for you.

If you have a migraine, however, this pose is best avoided.

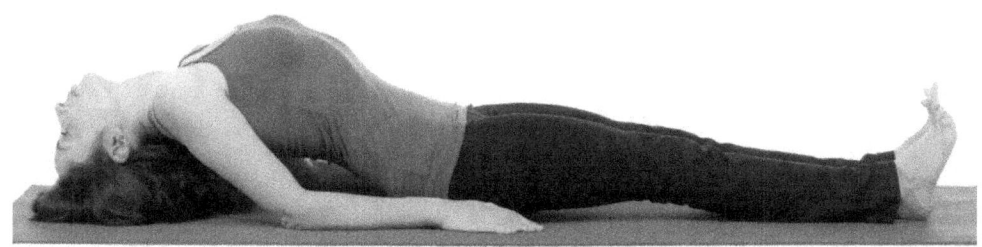

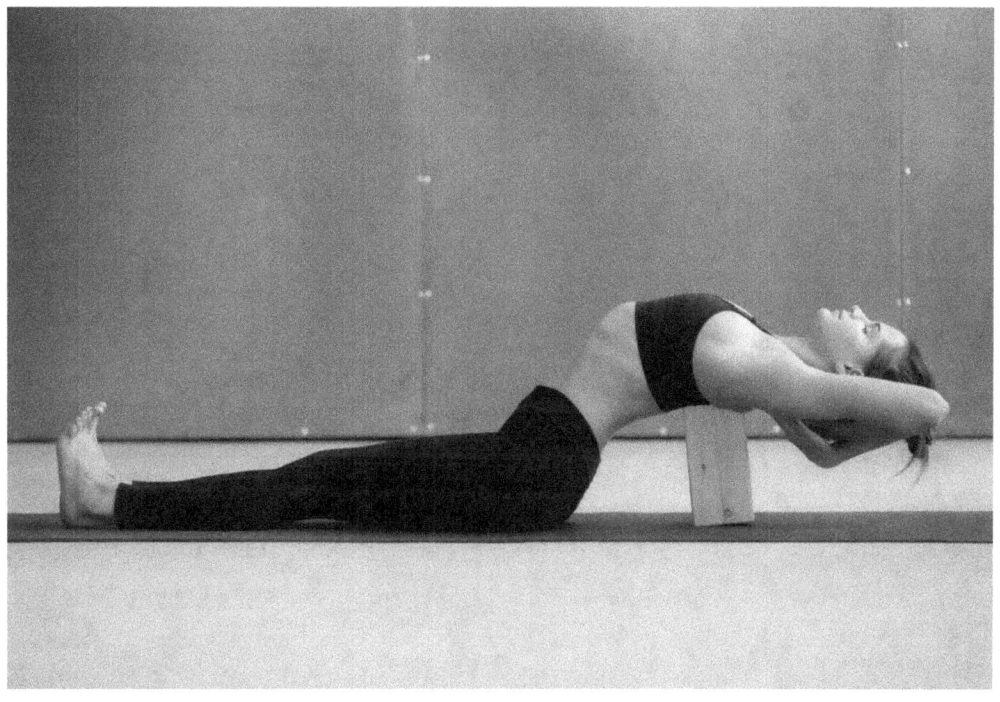

***Instructions***

1. Begin by lying on your back on your yoga mat with two blocks (or one block and a pillow) within arms' reach.
2. Inhale and lift your chest slightly. Insert a block on its side between your shoulder blades. Bend backwards over the block.
3. If this is too much for your neck, insert another block or a pillow beneath your head to take some of the pressure off.
4. Breathe deeply in this pose, allowing each breath to open the chest. Hold the posture for as long as needed.

# Cat and Cow Poses

*Sanskrit name: Marjaryasana/Bitilasana*

Cat/Cow Pose is actually two separate postures that are usually done in rounds, one after the other. Combined, they're a yoga classic; rarely will you leave a yoga class without doing Cat/Cow.

Cat Pose provides a stretch to the upper back, massages your internal organs, and allows the neck to hang loose and relax. Cow Pose stretches the front of the neck and broadens the chest, while likewise massaging your organs and spine.

This combination of poses gently warms up the neck and the spine, so it's best added in at the beginning of your yoga practice to release tension and prepare for more intense poses. The stretch to the front body and gentle massage of the stomach organs makes these poses a powerful tonic for digestive issues, so add the pair into your routine if you're struggling with autoimmune symptoms.

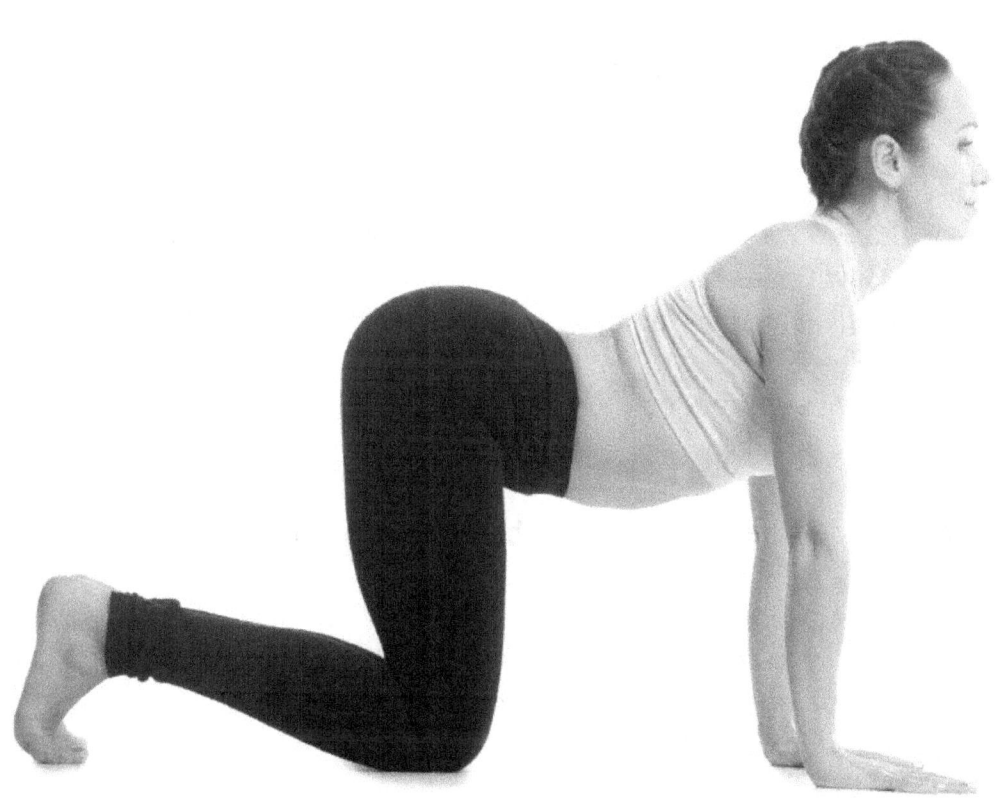

*Cow Pose*

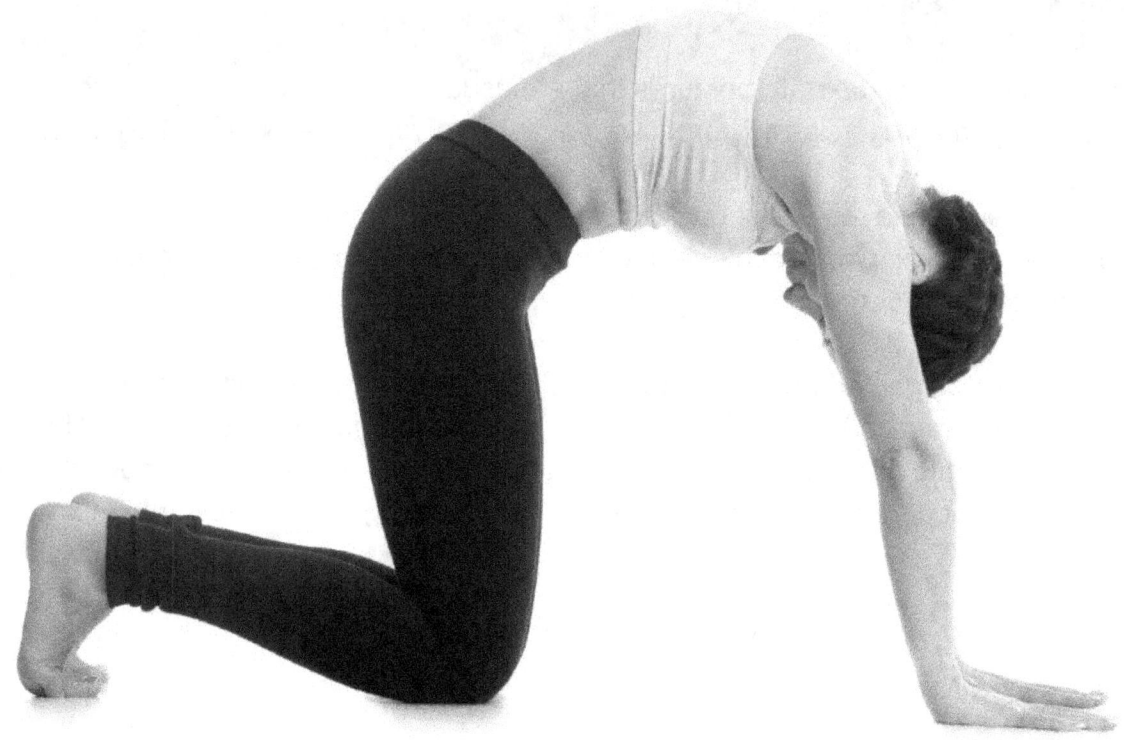

**Cat Pose**

## *Instructions*
1. Begin in Tabletop Pose.
2. On the inhale, arch your back downward, lift your chest and head, and lift your tailbone slightly to the sky. This is Cow Pose.
3. On the exhale, round your spine high, lowering your head and allowing it to dangle. Allow your neck to relax into Cat Pose.
4. Repeat this cycle as many times as needed.

## *Props*
1. If you are unable to rest on your knees, try adding a blanket or gel pads beneath them.

## *Modifications*
1. If your knees are still too sore, you can practice this pose standing up against a wall. Put your hands against the wall and mimic the movement of the postures.

# Rag Doll

*Sanskrit name: Baddha Hasta Uttanasana*

Rag Doll Pose, also known as Dangling Pose, is one of those super relaxing postures that's the perfect tonic for stress. This pose allows you to dangle your head to the ground, elongating your neck, and saying goodbye to tension in the neck and shoulders. It also provides a delicious stretch to your upper back and legs.

Because this pose is so simple, you can do it any time you need a break. This is the perfect pose to do behind your desk when your neck and back are hurting from looking down at your computer screen all day.

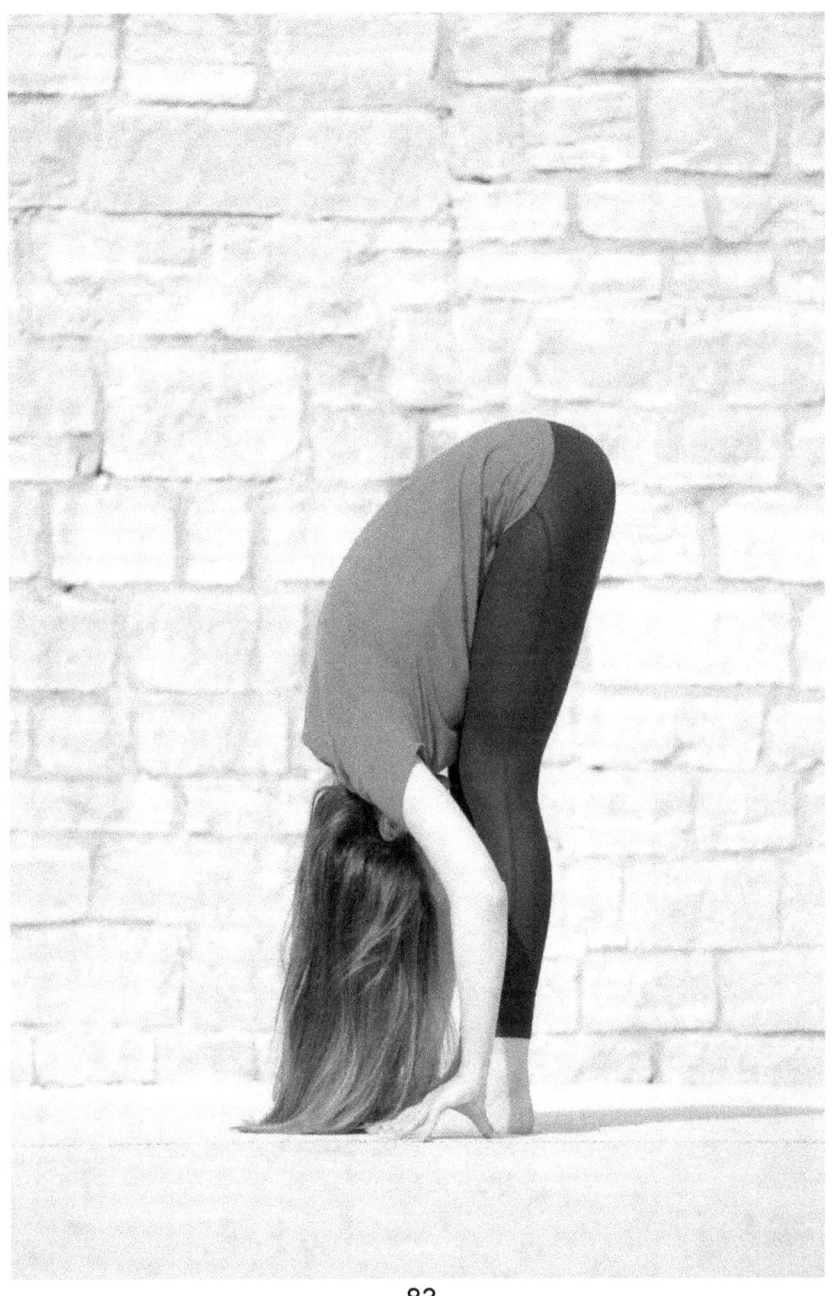

***Instructions***
1. Begin in Mountain Pose, with your feet hip distance apart.
2. Drape your entire body forward. Bend your knees slightly to reduce pressure on the knees. If your legs are very stiff, bend your knees as much as needed.
3. You may rest your hands on the ground, or grasp opposite elbows.
4. Allow your head to hang and your neck to become elongated.
5. Breathe in this pose for as long as is needed.

***Modifications***
1. To enhance the shoulder stretch, bend your knees until your chest is resting against your upper legs, then add a Hand Clasp behind your back.

# Standing Split

*Sanskrit name: Urdhva Prasarita Eka Padasana*

Standing Split is a kind of forward bend, so it allows your neck to release. This pose also stretches the entire leg and opens up the hips, while calming the mind. It's an inversion, making this a fantastic way to release tension from the entire body at the end of the day.

Standing Split also forces you to balance ever so slightly. Balancing poses provide a gentle workout to your core. Strengthening your core is key to preventing the injuries and lower back pain that come with arthritis and osteoporosis.

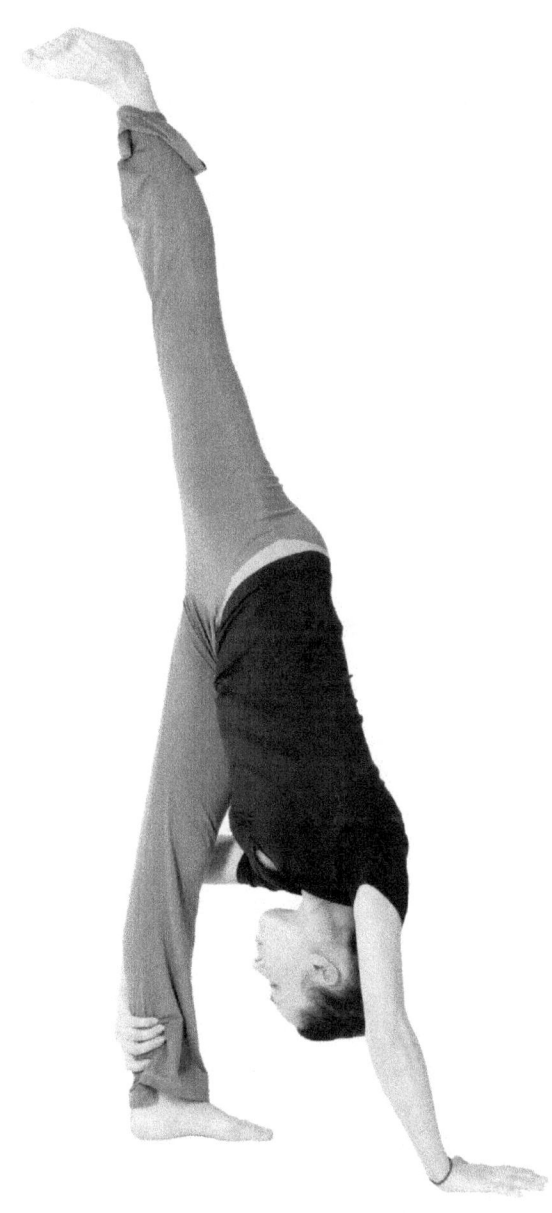

*Instructions*
1. Begin in Mountain Pose.
2. Bring your hands down to the mat and place your palms flat on the earth on either side of your right foot.
3. Spread your fingers for stability.
4. Lift your left leg towards the sky. You may only be able to get your leg up a few inches, but over time you'll be able to reach your leg higher.
5. Activate your leg and turn your toes down to the ground.
6. Ensure that your standing leg is not collapsing inwards.
7. Release your neck and allow gravity to gently pull on your head.
8. Breathe in this pose for as long as is comfortable, then repeat it on the other side.

*Props*
1. Support the lifted leg on a chair if this pose is too intense.
2. If your hands cannot reach the ground, place both hands on a block.

*Modifications*
1. Focus your gaze on a still point on the ground to help balance.
2. To deepen the pose and challenge your balance, grasp your hands around your standing ankle.

# Camel Pose

***Sanskrit name: Ustrasana***

Camel Pose can be pretty intense for beginners, so it's best to work your way up to this pose. Even if you've been doing yoga for a long time, Camel Pose is something you'll want to add in towards the end of your practice, once your neck and back have had the chance to warm up.

Camel Pose provides a deep stretch to the neck, throat, chest, shoulders, and stomach, so this pose can practically be a panacea for all of your body aches. The gentle stretch to the stomach also helps to alleviate the digestive discomfort caused by autoimmune disorders or heavy painkillers.

If you have a neck injury, knee pain, or a migraine, this pose should be skipped.

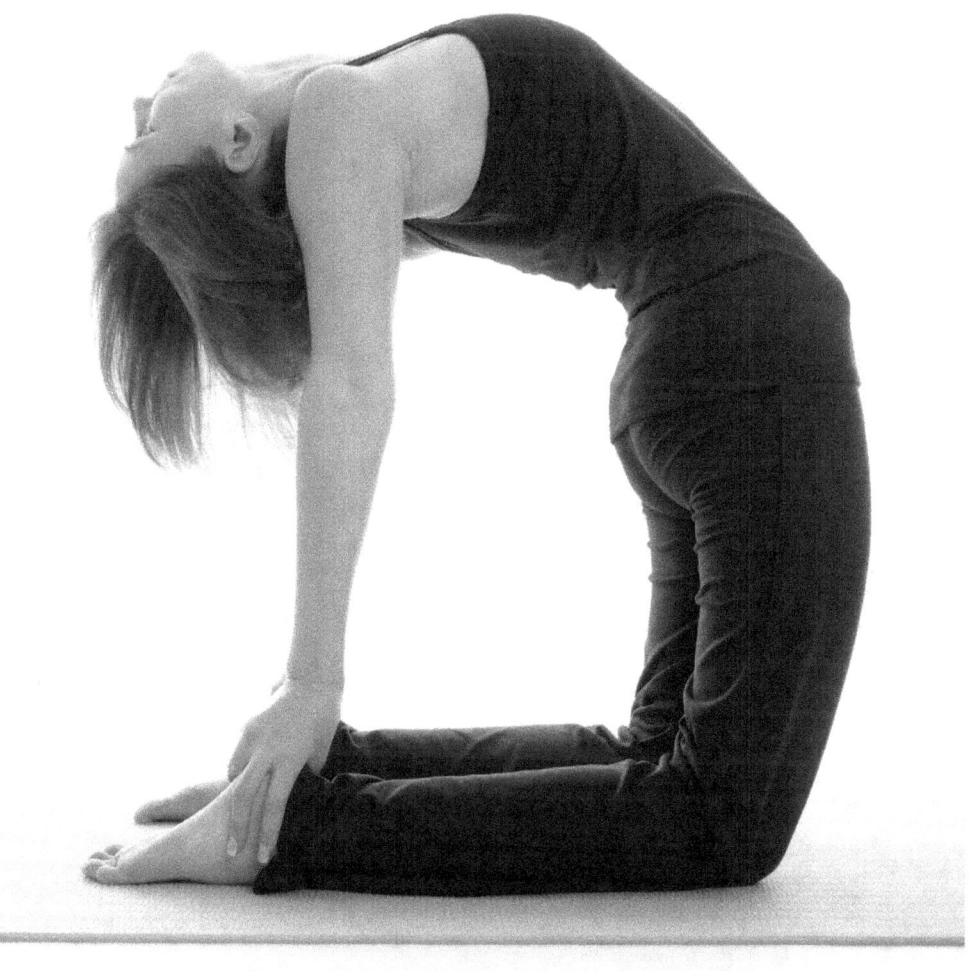

***Instructions***
1. Kneel on your mat with your knees hip distance apart.
2. Breathe in as you lengthen your entire body upwards, stretching the crown of your head towards the sky and elongating your neck.
3. Place your hands on your lower back, open your chest, lean your head backwards, and release your neck.
4. You can rest here or deepen the pose by reaching your hands further backwards to grab your heels.
5. Shut your eyes and breathe in a comfortable position for as long as needed, then release the pose.

***Props***
1. This pose might be tough on your knees. If you have sore knees, fold a blanket or your mat beneath them.

# Dolphin Pose

*Sanskrit name: Makarasana*

Like in Downward Facing Dog Pose, in Dolphin Pose your neck is able to hang freely, allowing gravity to deliver a gentle stretch to the neck. Dolphin Pose does, however, grant a more intense stretch to other parts of the body than Downward Facing Dog does. In Dolphin Pose, your upper back will also feel a major release, allowing your neck even more relief. If you sit behind a computer all day, you definitely need to add Dolphin Pose in to your routine to release the tension in your neck that makes arthritis pain so much worse.

A word of caution, this pose might be a little too intense if you have arthritis in your shoulders. Instead, work your way up to this pose and follow the instructions carefully to avoid injuring your shoulders.

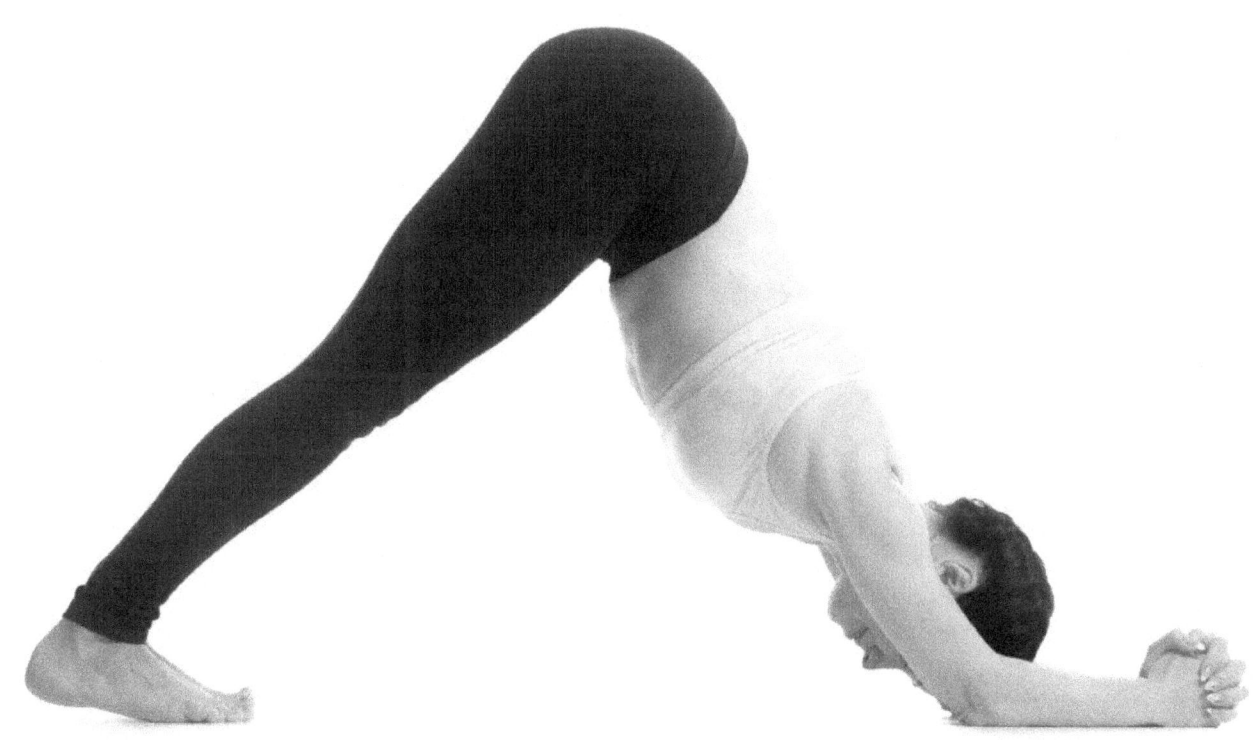

***Instructions***

1. From Tabletop Pose, lower onto your forearms. Your hands should be flat against your mat, with your fingers engaged and reaching out for stability.
2. Engage your arms and lift your hips until your hips are in the air and you are resting on the balls of your feet, like in Downward Facing Dog.
3. Make sure your shoulders are aligned with your elbows, and your elbows are not moving out to the side, to prevent shoulder injury.
4. Engage your legs to take the pressure off of your shoulders.
5. Take 5–10 breaths in this pose and allow your neck to dangle freely.
6. Slowly come down to your knees when you are ready to exit the pose.

# Upward Plank Pose

*Sanskrit name: Purvottanasana*

Not only does Upward Plank Pose help to release tension in the neck, it also opens up the entire front body, creating space where there used to just be tension. It's an excellent way to counterbalance sitting all day long. This pose does, however, provide more of a challenge than more restorative poses, so it's best to work your way up to this pose; do not begin with it right away.

If you're recovering from a back injury, this pose might not be the best for you. But if you want to create more flexibility in your back, Upward Plank Pose is a great way to prepare for more intense backbends.

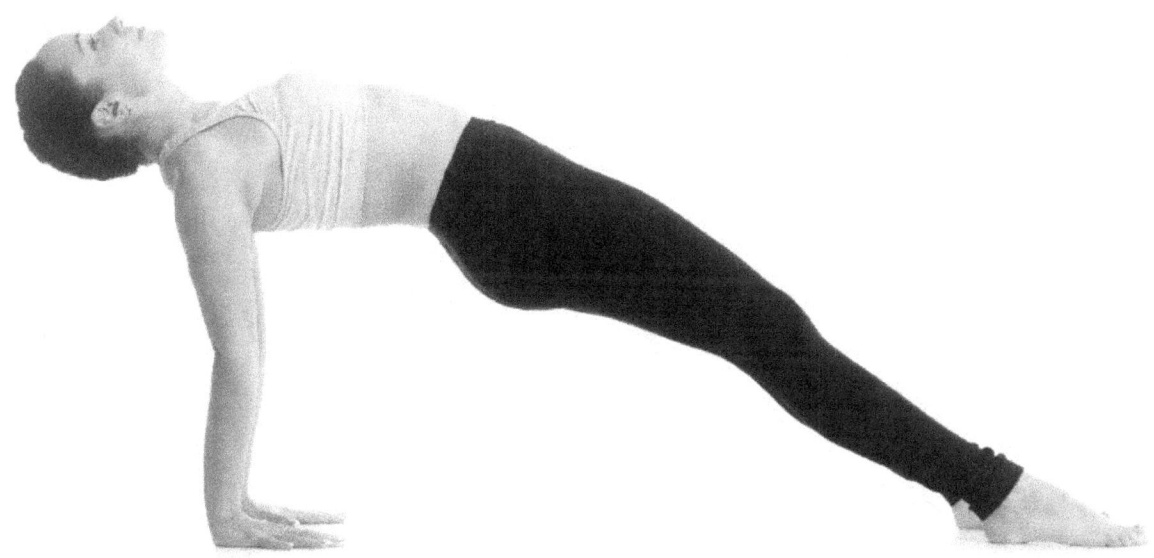

## Instructions
1. Begin sitting on the ground with your legs in front of you.
2. Your hands should be slightly behind your buttocks, no more than shoulder width apart. Your fingers should be pointing towards your feet.
3. Slowly begin to lift your hips with the soles of your feet planted on the ground. Your feet should be about hip width apart.
4. Lift your chest up and allow your neck to slowly release backwards.
5. Take 3–5 breaths in this pose and release.

## Modifications
1. If this pose is too difficult, you can practice Reverse Tabletop Pose instead. In Reverse Tabletop, you bend your knees at a 90-degree angle instead of fully extending your legs.
2. If this pose puts too much of a strain on your neck, practice with your head resting on a chair or against the wall.
3. If your wrists are too sore for this pose, just skip it and practice Cobra Pose or Sphinx Pose against a chair.

# Autoimmune Symptoms

Autoimmune disease in an umbrella term for diseases that cause the immune system to attack the body. Some of these diseases, like rheumatoid arthritis, reactive arthritis, and lupus, cause debilitating pain to the joints. Yoga can help you cope with this pain and bring flexibility to the inflamed joints.

Autoimmune diseases are also known to flare up during times of stress. This means reducing stress is one of the most important aspects to coping with an autoimmune disease. Luckily, yoga can help. The poses in this section are meant to bring the most gentle stretch to joints that are often hit hard by autoimmune disease, while helping to reduce stress and anxiety.

## Mountain Pose

*Sanskrit name: Tadasana*

Mountain Pose is one of the key poses in any yoga practice. It's so simple to do, you can do it even while you're waiting in line at the grocery store. This pose forces you to check in with your body and posture. Since the other joints in your body are connected to your spine, when your spine is out of alignment it can cause pain in many other joints. Mountain Pose is a perfect choice when you want to quickly correct your posture.

Because you focus on the feeling of your feet touching the earth, this pose is also very grounding, while the focus on the breath provides a de-stressing element you can add to your day anytime you want.

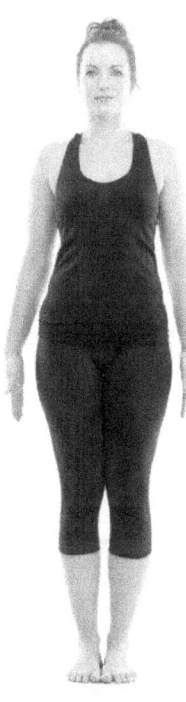

***Instructions***
1. Begin by standing upright. Check in with your feet. Balance your weight evenly on both feet and stretch out the toes.
2. Lift your kneecaps and your thighs. Activate your core, lift the pubis upwards, and lengthen the tailbone to the floor.
3. Widen your shoulder blades and move them down your back. Bring the neck straight and into alignment with the spine, and the chin parallel with the earth.
4. Breathe in the pose for as long as you'd like.

***Modifications***
1. To check your posture, you can practice doing this pose against a wall. Your shoulders should touch the wall, but the back of your head should not.

# Skull Shining Breath

*Sanskrit name: Kapalabhati*

Skull Shining Breath is a breathing technique that both calms and energizes the mind. It is also said to help the body eliminate toxins. Eliminating toxins is very important to ensuring that your immune system is functioning properly.

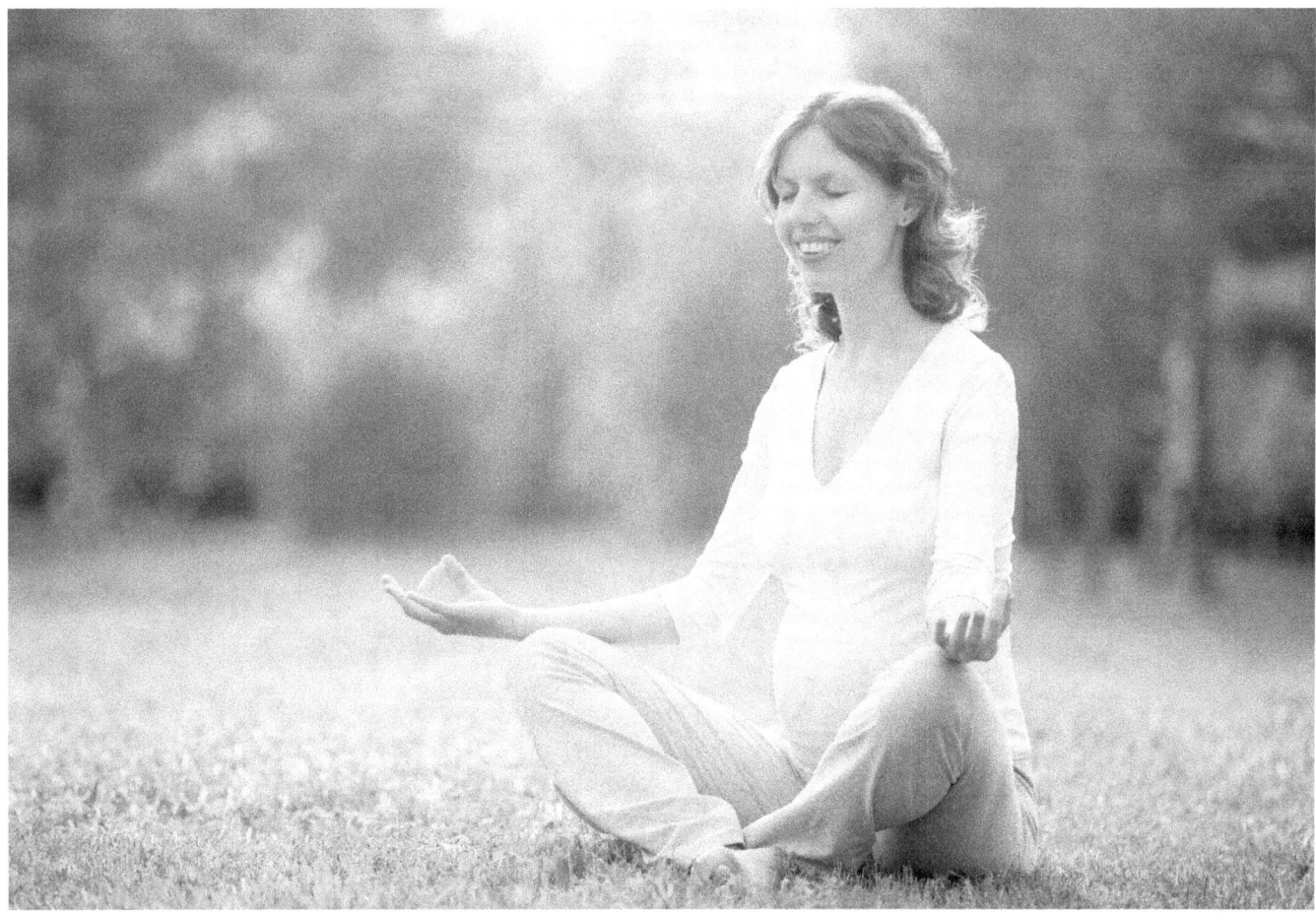

## Instructions
1. Sit comfortably in easy pose. Place the hands open, palms up on the knees.
2. Contract your lower belly to quickly force the air out of your lungs. Your lungs will fill with air automatically after the forceful contraction.
3. Repeat this motion about 30 times. Work your way up from there to more repetitions if you like how the breath makes you feel.

## Props
1. You may sit on a meditation pillow, if you prefer. You can also do this pose in a chair if sitting unsupported hurts your lower back.

## Modifications
1. It can be helpful to place one of your hands on your lower belly. This helps you to feel where the contraction should be coming from.

# Legs Up the Wall Pose

*Sanskrit name: Viparita Karani*

Legs Up the Wall Pose is pretty self-explanatory. This simple inversion pose is amazingly relaxing, especially for those who, like nurses and waitresses, spend much of the day on their feet. Since you're usually standing upright, fluids and toxins can get stuck in your legs. This pose helps to get everything moving.

When focusing on poses that relieve tension, we usually think of those that target the neck and shoulders, but your legs, buttocks, and feet tend to hold a lot of tension as well. This pose helps to diminish that, making it a fantastic pose to add to your nightly routine.

If you have an eye condition like glaucoma, inversion poses should be avoided.

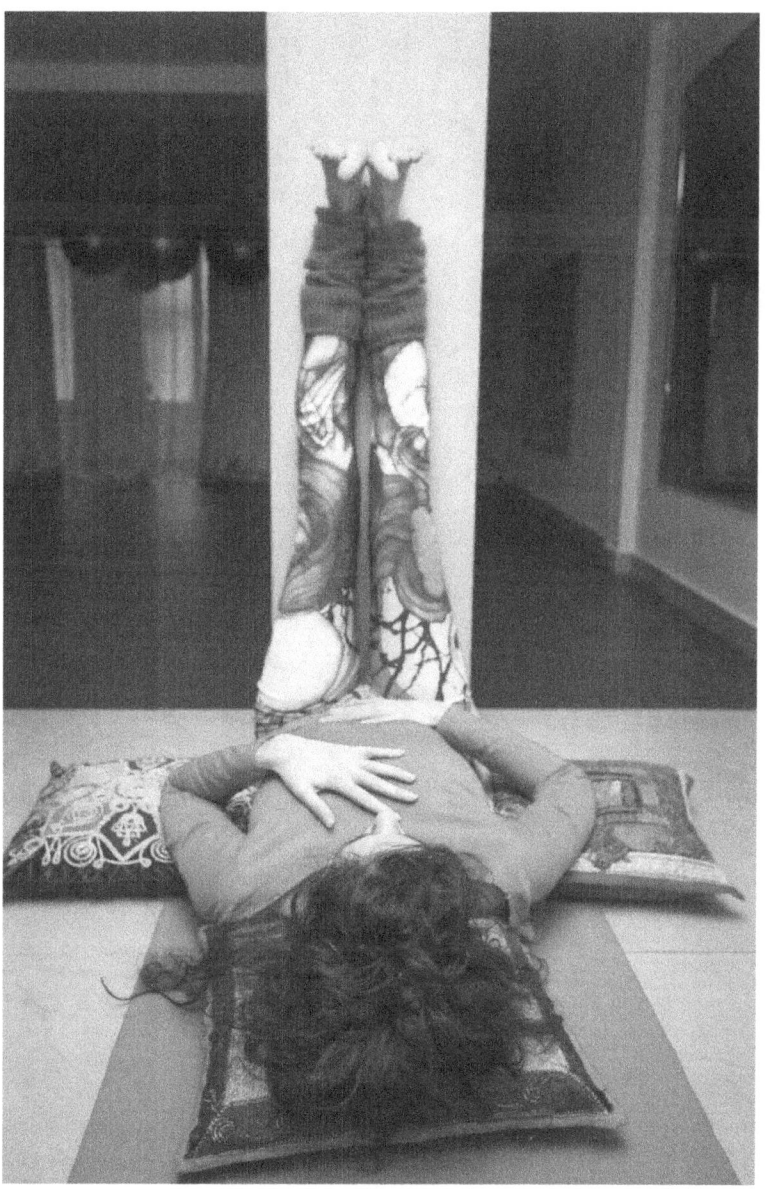

## Instructions

1. Begin by reclining on the floor near a wall. Inch your buttocks closer to the wall until they touch.
2. Move your legs up the wall until they are flat against the wall.
3. Hold this posture for as long as is comfortable. ten minutes would be a good time to aim for to feel the full stress-reducing benefits. Make sure not to turn your neck to the sides when in this pose.

## Props

1. To make this pose more restorative, place a block or bolster underneath your hips. You can also use a strap to bind your legs together so it's easier to keep them together.
2. For a more relaxing experience, you can also drape a washcloth over your eyes to block out light and distractions.

# Alternate Nostril Breathing

*Sanskrit name: Nadi Shodhana*

Autoimmune diseases are often accompanied by respiratory problems. Nadi Shodhana, the Sanskrit name for this breath, literally means *purifying the channel*. That's pretty much exactly what this pose does! Not only does this pose help to treat respiratory issues, while clearing mucus and toxins from the respiratory system, it's also deeply calming. Practice this pose next time you're congested or struggling with other respiratory issues.

If you're planning on entering a deeper meditation, this pose is a good way to prepare, so add this in before Savasana or another deep meditation.

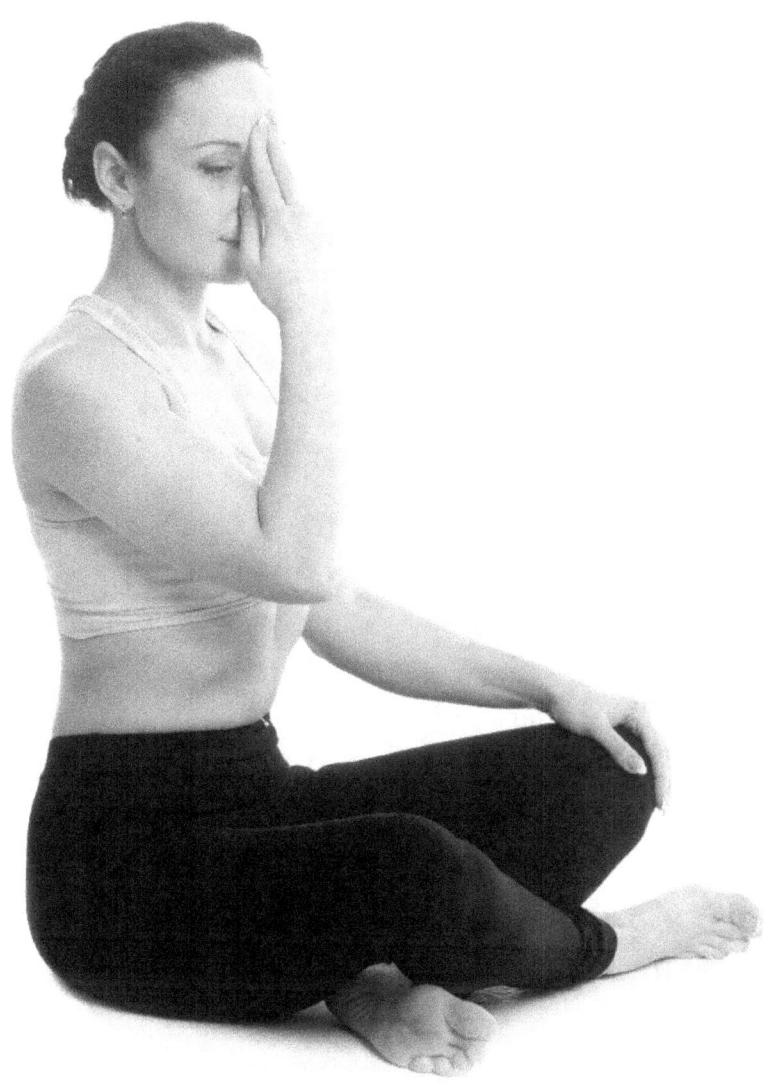

***Instructions***
1. Sit however is most comfortable for you, as long as your spine is straight and your shoulders are relaxed, but not slouched.
2. Place your right hand over your nose, with the index finger resting on your third eye, your thumb on your right nostril, and your ring finger over your left nostril.
3. Close your eyes.
4. Use your thumb to close your right nostril and inhale deeply through your left nostril.
5. Hold your breath at the top of the breath while you use your ring finger to block off the left nostril.
6. Remove your thumb from your right nostril and exhale. Repeat as many times as needed.

***Props***
1. A good prop for this pose is a meditation pillow to sit on, but you can also sit in a chair if you need back support.
2. Do not practice this breath without a tissue at hand, because it tends to get mucus moving through the respiratory system.

# Staff Pose

*Sanskrit name: Dandasana*

This pose is called Staff Pose because your spine should be straight and firm like a staff. Staff Pose brings strength to the hips and core, while delivering a stretch to your shoulders and chest. Practicing this pose on a regular basis will help you to develop better posture, leading to a reduction in body aches and pains, especially in the back and neck. It also will bring a much-needed stretch into your often forgotten ankles.

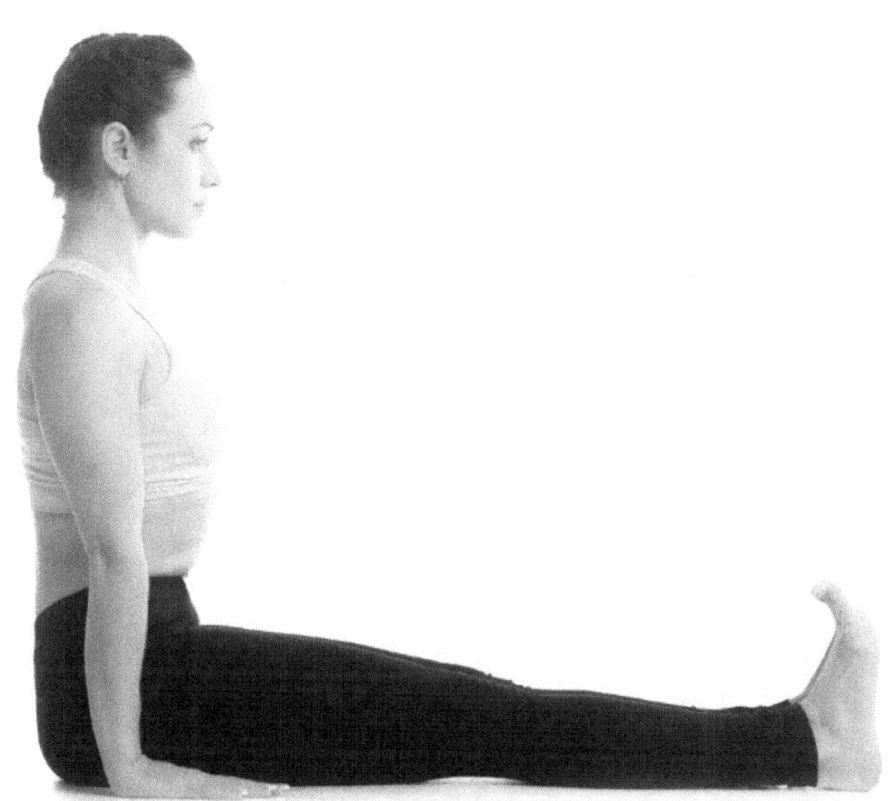

## Instructions
1. Sit on your yoga mat with your legs straight in front of you.
2. Check in with your body to make sure you are evenly distributing your weight through your sitting bones and that they are firmly grounded on the earth.
3. Flex your feet, pushing through the heels.
4. Activate your legs.
5. Lengthen your entire upper body, moving your crown towards the sky.

6. Check in to make sure your neck is directly over your tailbone and your jaw is parallel with the earth. Make sure your shoulders are not moving upwards towards your ears. Instead, coax them down your back.
7. Place your hands, palms down besides your hips.
8. Take about 10 breaths in this pose, or as many as are needed to feel relaxed.

**Props**
1. If your hands do not reach the ground, place a block beneath each hand.

# Restorative Reclining Bound Angle Pose

*Sanskrit name: Supta Baddha Konasana*

Bound Angle Pose might just be the most relaxing yoga pose ever, but adding these restorative elements makes it even better. Reducing autoimmune symptoms is all about reducing stress, so this pose can be a really powerful addition into your healing toolkit. Not only is this pose deeply relaxing and grounding, it also helps to relieve digestive discomfort, opens up the chest, and provides a stretch to the hips.

Sometimes traditional bound angle can be painful if you're dealing with low back pain. It can also be tough on the knees and some people find the hip stretch a little too intense. The restorative version uses props to reduce or eliminate all of these issues. Since this is a restorative pose, with the right props you can hang out in this pose for up to 20–30 minutes.

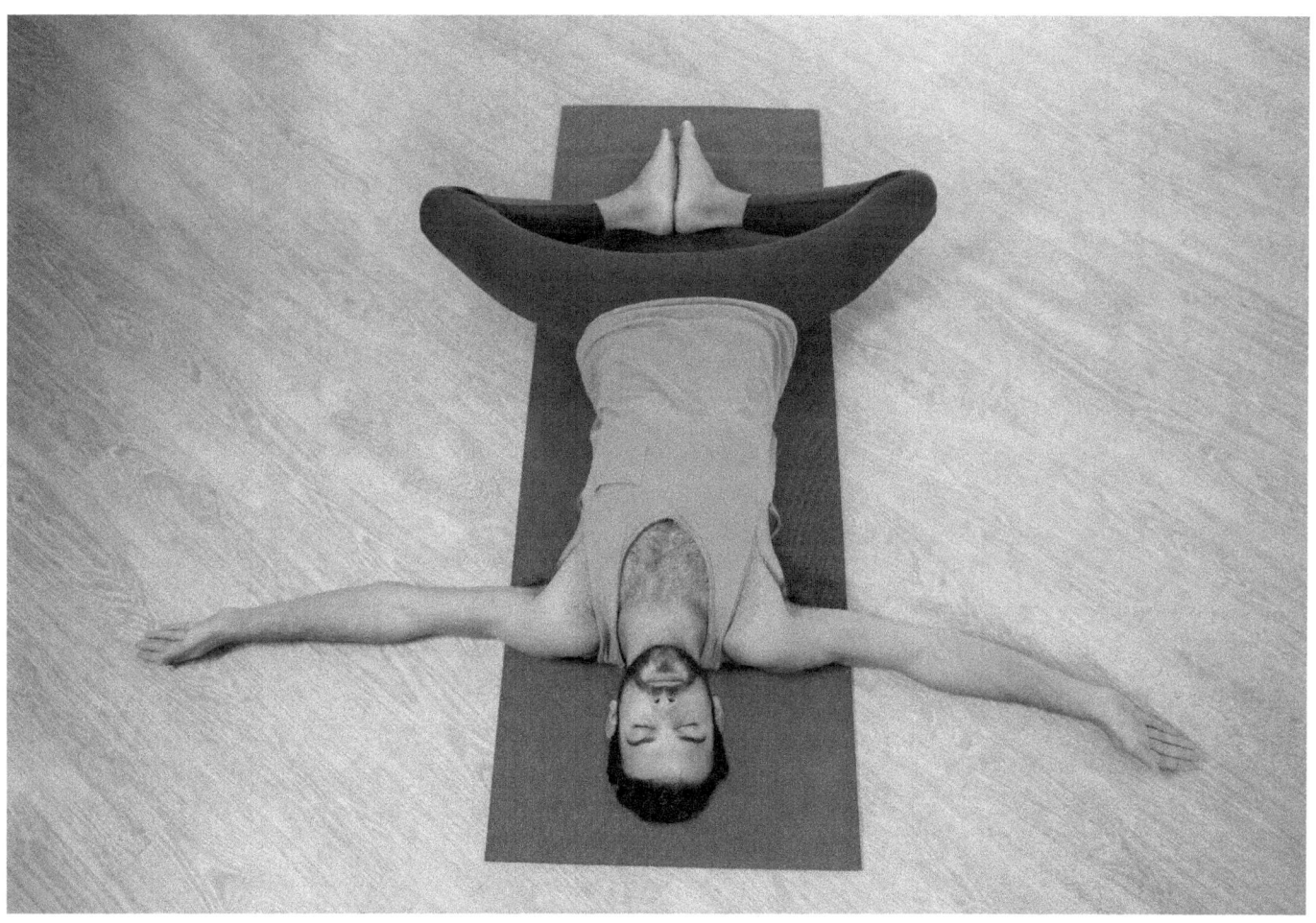

## Instructions

1. Recline on your back and bring the soles of your feet together. Spread your arms out to your sides. This is simple Reclined Bound Angle.
2. To make this pose restorative, add a bolster under your back and head. This will prevent lower back pain and any strain to your neck.
3. Add any other props you may need, and breathe to open the chest. Breathe in this pose as long as you like.

## Props

1. A bolster under the back adds the restorative element.
2. If you'd like to stay in this pose for a long time, it's recommended that you place blocks or bolsters under your knees to prevent the stretch in your hips from becoming too intense.
3. For more relaxation, place a washcloth over your eyes to block out light and distractions.

# Corpse Pose

*Sanskrit name: Savasana*

It is often said that every other yoga posture is leading up to Savasana. This simple pose has been called the most difficult pose in the entire yoga canon. But why? It's because so many people find resting and stillness nearly impossible. If you can manage to relax and let go of your thoughts in this pose, you'll be treated with some deep meditation, or at least a few very restful minutes.

You can stay in this pose pretty much as long as is comfortable for you. It's best done at the end of your practice. Because it's so relaxing, this is a great choice for a posture to do just before bed. There are many props and modifications you can add to make this pose as comfortable as possible for you.

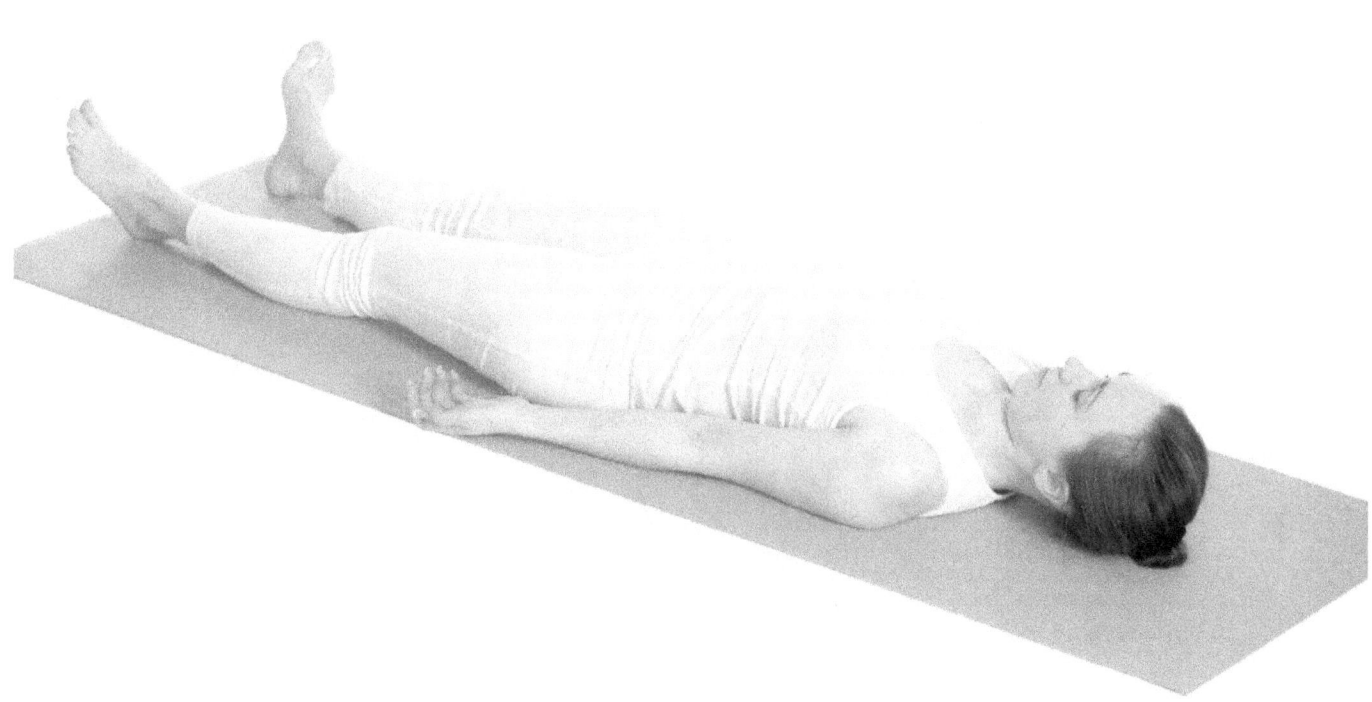

## Instructions
1. Recline on the ground, with your arms comfortably draped at your sides, palms facing upwards.
2. Allow your feet to turn outwards slightly.
3. Take three deep cleansing breaths, then breathe naturally.

4. Allow your mind to become quiet. Gently let go of any thoughts that pass through your mind.
5. Remain in this pose as long as is comfortable.

## *Props*
1. If you are worried about bringing tension to your neck and head, place a folded blanket beneath them.
2. To relax the legs and lower back, place a chair in front of you. Lift your legs up and rest them across the seat of the chair.

## *Modifications*
1. To protect your lower back from strain, feel free to practice this pose with your knees bent and your feet flat on the floor.

# Parting Words and The Yoga Lifestyle

If you've been enjoying your yoga journey, and we hope you have been, then you might want to learn more about the underlying principles of a yoga as a lifestyle.

### *Ahimsa*
This is the first, and the biggest, yoga principle. It means "not to injure," and it applies in many important areas in our lives:
- How we treat all living beings
- How we treat ourselves, in mind and body
- How we think, and what we dedicate our thoughts to
- How we talk, and what we talk about
- How, and what, we put into our bodies

This principle is about the virtue of gentleness, nonviolence, and compassion. Because all things have a little bit of divine energy, then to hurt one thing is to hurt all things, including yourself.

### *Satya*
Satya refers to honesty, but it teaches that we do so without ever having the intent to hurt anyone. We speak honestly, but diplomatically.

### *Asteya*
This principle teaches that we only take what we need, leaving the rest for others.

### *Asparigraha*
Related to Asteya, this is the virtue of living simply, and not requiring too much. Minimalism is more compatible with a yogic lifestyle.

### *Brahmacharya*
Be steadfast and loyal in all aspects of your life – your relationships, your job, and all your dealings.

These principles are intended to lead the practitioner to a life of lasting happiness. It's simple, but it has many layers. You find peace by learning to control your thinking, and when you are the master of your own mind, you choose to live in the light of peace and happiness.

Namasté.

You might also enjoy:

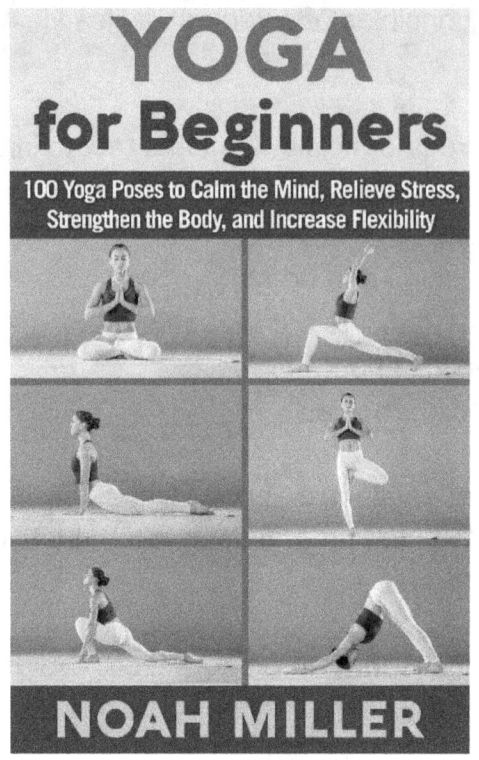

**Image Credits**

*Bharadvaja's Twist*
By Mr. Yoga (http://mryoga.com/seated-yoga-poses/) [CC BY-SA 4.0 (https://creativecommons.org/licenses/by-sa/4.0)], via Wikimedia Commons

www.ingramcontent.com/pod-product-compliance
Lightning Source LLC
Chambersburg PA
CBHW062219220526
45471CB00009B/3262